THE OPERATING MANUAL FOR GREAT HEALTH

How to Achieve Peak Wellness and Find Your True Self

BENJAMIN T. MUELLER

As I always tell my students, no matter how much you know about a topic, there is always more to learn. Ultimately, we learn from our past experiences, interactions with others, and perhaps our own research. Without a doubt, I owe everything that I know to another person.

There are many people who played a major role in the development of my life and this book. I could not possibly mention everyone, but I would like to thank the following:

To all my past teachers at Sheboygan Lutheran High School, Horace Mann Middle School, and James Madison Elementary School, not only did you teach me the skills needed to be successful, but you inspired me to be the best that I can be. Despite the challenges I faced in school, you encouraged me to keep my head up high and keep moving forward.

I would like to thank all of the citizens of Sheboygan, Wisconsin. I believe there is a lot of truth in the phrase, "It takes a village to raise a child." Sheboygan was the perfect city to grow up in and learn about life. I will always cherish my memories of Lake Michigan, refereeing in the Sheboygan Soccer League, and the many miles of running throughout the streets of Sheboygan. To put it best, it does not get better than Sheboygan, Wisconsin.

Next, I would like to thank the citizens of Dekalb County. When I moved here in 2006, I did not know a single person. You all welcomed me with open arms, and I have met so many wonderful people.

Special thank you to my foreword writers, Dr. Michael Olpin and Dr. Jasbir Kocher. I have learned so much about health and optimal thinking from both of you over the years. Your forewords mean the world to me, and I was honored to have both of you on board.

I must thank all of my past students for their efforts, interest, curiosity, questions, and desire to learn over the years. After being a wellness educator for ten years, I have taught over 500 students. Your interests, curiosity, and questions have extended my knowledge on various topics.

I would like to thank all of my past chiropractors. Not only have you kept my spine and nervous system in great condition, but you have extended my knowledge in virtually every area of health. In particular, I would like to thank Dr. Brent Maxwell and Dr. Jessica Melby.

Special thanks to editor Kathryn F. Galán for your patience and guidance in the development of this book.

Last, but certainly not least, I would like to thank my parents. Thank you for always believing in me and encouraging me to look beyond my comfort zone. There are many times when I doubted myself and you gave me that extra push that I needed.

CONTENTS

Foreword

GOOD AND LONG-LASTING health is not rocket science. It's true, each of us is different—there is no such thing as one-size-fits-all when we try to figure out which behaviors lead to which health outcomes. But we know that healthier people consistently do certain things in certain ways; those things they do create sufficient balance so the body/mind can heal itself—and improve.

With so much health information available "out there," it is easy to be confused. What works? What doesn't?

Ben has done the heavy lifting for the rest of us. He has figured out what the experts know and what the research suggests, and put that knowledge into a very interesting book that is packed with useful health information. Essentially, Ben takes us by the hand and carefully walks with us in a better direction, health-wise.

There's a really cool saying that goes something like this: Good health—a thousand desires; bad health—one desire. To me, good health means being able to do the things I choose to do at the level I choose to do them. If I can know what works to keep me in a healthy state, then I'm free to do everything else I want to do.

Do "bad" things happen with our health that seem unavoidable? Sure. But if I can tip the scales in my favor, I can go a long way in preventing problems from happening in the first place. To me that's the smartest thing, and it is what Ben has nicely done. This book is a simple, succinct, and practical approach to lifelong wellness.

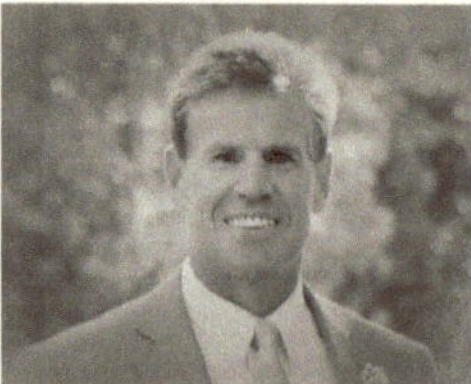

Dr. Michael Olpin, Professor, WSU
Director, WSU Stress Relief Center
https://stressmanagementplace.com

Foreword

100% HEALTH equals 100% FUNCTION.

Let me ask you all a simple yet PROFOUND question—when your health is at its worst, are you able to do the things you love to do or be with the people you love to be around in the best way possible?

Briefly look back to a time when you were feeling sick and/or unhappy, and you may recall this challenging time and perhaps the negatively charged feeling you may have experienced.

On the flip side of the coin—when you are feeling happy and healthy, you are most capable of doing the things you love to do and can be the best version of yourself with the people you love to be around, right? In other words, when you are healthy, you allow yourself the opportunity to function at your best; you can push yourself beyond your limitations by reaching toward your fullest potential. The longer I'm in practice, the more authentic this statement becomes—100% FUNCTION equals 100% HEALTH.

As a chiropractic physician, I am humbly given the opportunity and the privilege to serve others, propelling them to reach their highest potential. I do this by delivering a specific and intentional force to their spine, freeing up any interference to their nervous system, and allowing their body to tap into its innate ability to heal itself—from the inside-out, literally.

A classic example of this is when we get a paper cut. We do not have to *tell* our body to heal itself. Our innate consciousness sends the message from our brain above, down through our spinal cord and nerves, to our cells, allowing the body to heal itself from the inside out. This concept is termed "above-down, inside-out."

It's important to keep in mind that I, the practitioner, am not doing the healing; I am merely delivering an intentional force to the spine, allowing the nervous system do what it is designed to do—allowing us to function fully.

On March 6, 2017, I had the honor of meeting Ben. And to say the least, Ben is genuine and one-of-a-kind. It's not surprising to me that he is striving to do more than just be an in-classroom teacher. He is also a coach, an avid runner, and an inspiring author.

I love the idea of this book because it is tying together all of the vital options that complete the health puzzle we term "wellness." I am proud of you, Ben. And I am honored to continue serving you and riding alongside you throughout your wellness journey. God bless you, Ben, and keep *moving* forward, my friend.

Namaste.

Dr. Jasbir Singh Kocher, D.C.

BEN MUELLER

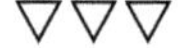

Introduction

MY MOTIVATION to write this book began on a typical Sunday, while I was grocery shopping. As I was waiting in line to check out, I noticed the surplus of "so-called" health magazines by the counter. As I looked at the magazines and the "air-brushed" photos on the front cover, I was reminded of how poorly Americans truly understand health.

We are constantly bombarded with messages such as "low fat," "lose 10 pounds in 10 days," "sweat off 15 pounds," "look 5 years younger," etc. Of course, all of this is nothing more than propaganda by multi-million-dollar industries trying to take advantage of people's desperation to improve their health and get them to bite on something that simply won't work. At least, not in the long term!

What bothers me the most about this is that good health does not need to be rocket science. In fact, it simply is not! Let me repeat that. Good health is NOT rocket science! One more time: good health is NOT rocket science! If you are looking for that special diet, special exercise program, or magic pill that will suddenly flip your health around, it is not out there. Sorry to be the first one to break it to you.

What does work is lifestyle changes. We need to get back to the very basics. Everyone needs to have an honest conversation with themselves about their lifestyle habits and the impact they are having on our overall health. Are you exercising? How is your nutrition? Are you putting any toxins in your body regularly? Are you getting enough quality sleep each night? These are the questions we need to be asking ourselves. That is, we need to put away these *fad* magazines and celebrity diet-advice books, or whatever it is you are reading, and go back to square one.

Now, I know what you're thinking:

"What gives you the right to write a health book? You're not a doctor! You're not a celebrity! You're not a famous athlete! You do not have a doctoral degree in health!"

Oh please! You do not need to be a doctor to know how to live healthy. According to the National Center for Biotechnical Information, the average doctor has a life expectancy five years less than the average person! (No offense to the doctors out there.) Also, most of the celebrities and athletes who wrote a book probably just had a ghostwriter author it for them, anyways.

As an endurance athlete, my interest in health began with the link between health and performance. I quickly discovered that the healthier you are, the better you perform, not only in running but in life.

Now, back to this book! If you are looking for a book that is complicated and requires an advanced degree to understand it, then this book is not for you. In writing this book, my goal was to keep it basic and easy to understand. My goal is to motivate you to make healthier choices and provide you with the information needed to get started.

The contents of this book merge what I have learned regarding health over the years from a variety of sources. It is written in an easy-to-read and accessible format, divided in short sections. You can read the entire book straight through or refer to the Table of Contents for a specific section or topic.

If you have any questions, please contact me at Ben.Mueller7@aol.com.

With that, I wish you happy reading and learning. Here's to a healthier you and a better life!

Did you know?

The average person who starts a fad diet gains five pounds a year later. Fad diets don't work!!

The Dalai Lama, when asked what surprised him most about humanity, answered, "Man, because he sacrifices his health in order to make money. Then he sacrifices money to recuperate his health. And then he is so anxious about the future that he does not enjoy the present; the result being that he does not live in the present or the future. He lives as if he is never going to die, then dies having never really lived."

Health Crisis

WHEN YOU LOOK at the average adult, what do you see in their physical health? How about their mental health? Here are some things you may see amongst many adults in our society:

- ➢ Smokes tobacco products
- ➢ Is overweight or obese
- ➢ Relies on medications to get through a day
- ➢ Has difficulty walking
- ➢ Is in a lot of pain and relies on opiate pain killers
- ➢ Addicted to processed food
- ➢ Under a lot of stress
- ➢ Gets easily angered and upset
- ➢ Is in a state of depression, without a positive outlook on life.

Now, ask yourself, is that what you want to see for yourself?

Sure, there are a lot of people who seem to be healthy, full of energy, and in good spirits. On the other hand, though, *most* Americans do not fit in that category.

For example, many Americans rely on prescription medications to control symptoms that result from poor health choices. Furthermore, smoking continues to be the leading cause of preventable death in the United States, and obesity is not far behind in second place.

The top two causes of death in the United States are heart disease and cancer, respectively. Other diseases that continue to cripple Americans include diabetes, osteoporosis, arthritis, emphysema, and hypertension. For the first time ever, the younger generation of children is predicted to have a life expectancy less than their parents'. Childhood obesity is on the rise, and early signs of heart disease are beginning to show in children as young as eight years old.

Living in a developed nation like the United States does have its advantages in terms of medical care, vaccinations, sanitary conditions, and access to clean food that the poorer nations don't have. While America has the best medicine and medical technology in the world, United States citizens have a shorter life expectancy than citizens in other countries. The United States of America ranks worst of all the developed nations in each of the following:

- ✓ Percent of citizens obese or overweight
- ✓ Percent of citizens diagnosed with a mental disease
- ✓ Number of homicides per capita
- ✓ Percent of citizens living in poverty
- ✓ Percent of people who are homeless
- ✓ Percent of citizens incarcerated
- ✓ Highest infant mortality rate
- ✓ Overall life expectancy
- ✓ Percent of people addicted to an illegal drug
- ✓ Percent of people addicted to opiates
- ✓ Highest rate of teenage pregnancies

✓ Highest rate of people being diagnosed with a sexually transmitted disease including HIV

These facts above are very sad, especially given the fact that America spends more than twice on health care per person than any other developed nation. No doubt, the results should be much better than this.

###

Did you know?

The United States spent $9,507 on health per person in 2017, which is the highest of any country. Not only that, but this is more than twice the average of all the developed countries. Despite this, the United States has the worst health outcomes of all the developed nations. The U.S. is also the only developed country in the world that does not have guaranteed health care for all citizens.

Five Essentials to Health

WHAT ARE THE behaviors that lead to excellent health and peak performance? What do people who are free of disease, full of high energy, ambitious, are clear thinkers, and have a positive outlook have in common? What choices do they make that lead to excellent health? Are they just lucky? Or are they doing something that the majority of people are not doing?

Most likely, people who have reached a level of excellent health are doing well in each of the five essentials to excellent health.

There are five essentials needed for excellent health and wellness. I like to think of the five essentials as the blueprint to excellent health. Each of the essentials is equally important for maintaining proper body function and a healthy mindset.

On a regular basis, a person seeking excellent health should reflect on each of these essentials and should strive to do their absolute best in each essential. If any of the essentials is lacking, they should seek to improve it. The five essentials to excellent health are:

1. **Nutrition**: Providing your body with the right nutrients through eating mostly whole, nutrient-dense foods.
2. **Exercise**: Staying active through regular physical activity involving the proper balance of all the fitness components.
3. **Sleep**: Getting the proper rest and recovery that your body needs every night.
4. **Minimizing toxins**: Avoiding chemicals and substances that disrupt the flow of your body.
5. **Mindset**: Having a positive mindset, outlook, and thought process.

Again, each of the essentials is important, and if one of the essentials is lacking, it can have a severe negative effect on your overall wellness.

For example, if one exercises a lot and consumes a poor diet, their overall health will suffer despite all the exercise that they do. The exercise may help keep some of the physical symptoms away, such as high blood pressure and obesity, but the poor nutrition will eventually catch up with the person.

It is very important not to rely on just a few of the essentials to keep you healthy, but to stay strong in each essential. The next section summarizes the keys to staying strong in each of the five essentials and provides a good checklist for you to assess your current health behaviors.

The 5 Health Essentials of Health (Blueprint to Excellent Health)

Essential 1: Nutrition

A. Consume foods that are closer to their natural state and less processed.

B. Aim to consume 51% or more of your foods raw. (Fresh veggies, fruit, seeds, nuts, mushrooms, etc.)

C. Eliminate processed foods and replace them with whole foods as much as possible.

D. It is not about dieting. It is about a lifestyle!

E. Super foods: beans, berries, onions, seeds, mushrooms, and greens

F. Think *QUALITY*, *QUANTITY*, and *VARIETY* when it comes to consuming a balanced diet. Get lots of colors of plant-based foods!

G. It is not about calories or nutrient isolation! Don't be fooled by industry! Whole foods fill you up and make you feel full.

H. Drink lots of water. Water helps your body detoxify and many other things. Drink water!

I. Remember: all foods have protein. All plant-based foods are about ten percent protein.

J. Fat is not bad! Healthy fats include fish, nuts, seeds, omega 3s, flax seed, avocados, etc.

K. Get plenty of vitamin D3 and omega 3s!

Essential 2: Exercise

A. Exercise optimizes your oxygen intake and helps your body to produce muscle.

B. The best exercise is HIIT (High Intensity Interval Training). This type of exercise actually increases your human growth hormone and endorphins, lowers blood sugar, increases muscle mass, lowers heart rate, and improves stamina.

C. Any exercise is good! Whatever you like to do! Moving large muscles is a great way to improve mood and manage stress.

D. Make sure to take time to recover. The body gets stronger during recovery!

Essential 3: Sleep

A. Keep a consistent sleep schedule.

B. Get seven to nine hours of sleep per night.

C. During sleep, your brain and body repair. It is critical!

D. Chronic sleep deprivation can lead to an increased risk for all diseases. It lowers your immune system! You get an immune boost during sleep!

Essential 4: Minimize Toxins

A. By minimizing your exposure to toxins, you are keeping your body free from the unknown risks that are associated with trying to cover up symptoms such as headaches, weight gain, nausea, and depression.

B. Read labels and do your research! The chemicals added to processed foods, skin products, makeup, and cleaning products could potentially harm our bodies. Do your research, and choose products that have less of these toxins in them.

C. Do not smoke or use e-cigarettes! Smoking leads to exposing yourself to thousands of known carcinogens.

D. Limit alcohol consumption! Alcohol can harm your liver, brain, and body. Do not drink if you are under the age of twenty-one.

E. Do your research! Read, ask questions, get a variety of opinions, and dig for the information. The information is there! You need to want to get to it.

Essential 5: Maximized Mind

A. Your actions will always follow your beliefs. Everything starts with the mind!

B. Get rid of all negative thoughts immediately. They are road blocks! *THINK POSITVE*!

C. Find whatever beliefs you have about yourself that are preventing you from getting where you want to be, and eliminate them.

D. Visualize success—the subconscious mind cannot tell the difference between imagination and reality.

E. Your beliefs about yourself can be changed through constant positive self-talk.

F. Determine your purpose in life. Turn your passions into your life!

G. Remember: *you* decide if you enter the "flight or fight" mode. Don't get stressed out over the small stuff!

###

Did you know?

Dr. Dean Ornish has been able to heal patients with advanced heart disease without medication. He uses a vegetarian diet, stress reduction, and light exercise to help the patient's body heal itself. Check out his book called *UnDo It: How Simple Lifestyle Changes Can Reverse Most Chronic Diseases.*

Health Survey

The following is a short survey you can take to assess your current choices and the effects they may have on your overall health.

###

1. How many cups of water do you drink per day?

A) 0-2

B) 3-4

C) 5-6

D) 7 or more

2. How many servings of fruit and vegetables do you eat per day?

A) 0-1

B) 2-3

C) 4-5

D) 6 or more

3. How many cans of soda do you drink per week?

A) 10 or more

B) 5-9

C) 2-4

D) 1 or less

4. How many packages of unhealthy snacks do you eat per day? (potato chips, candy bars, etc.)

A) 5 or more

B) 4-5

C) 2-3

D) 1 or less

5. How many minutes of exercise do you get per day?

A) 0-14

B) 15-30

C) 31-59

D) More than 60

6. How many hours per day do you spend watching TV, playing video games, or in front of a computer?

A) More than 4

B.) 3-4 hrs.

C) 1-2 hrs.

D) Less than1 hr.

7. How many times per week do you work on your flexibility through stretching, yoga, or some other means?

A) 0

B) 1

C) 2

D) 3 or more

8. How many hours of sleep do you get on a weeknight?

A) 4 or less

B) 5-6

C) 7

D) 8 or more

9. How many hours do you spend on your cell phone or watching TV while lying in bed?

A) More than 3

B) About 2

C) Less than 1 hr.

D. 0

10. When you get extremely stressed out, do you have "go to" activities you do?

A) Never

B) Sometimes

C) Most of the time

D) Always

11. Do you spend time daily planning and prioritizing your days?

A) Never

B) Sometimes

C) Most of the time

D.) Always

12. In general, what is your attitude about approaching new challenging tasks?

A) Rather not try

B) Try and give up quick

C) Try, but eventually give up

D) Will reach goal

Scoring

How many Ds? _____ x 4 = _____

How many Cs? _____ x 3 = _____

How many Bs? _____ x 2 = _____

How many As? _____ x 1 = _____

###

Totals Results

42 or more: You are currently taking many measures to live a healthy life style. Keep it up!

36-41: Great job! You are doing a lot to keep yourself healthy. There are a few areas you could sharpen up on.

30-35: Your health habits are decent. Some changes are necessary to reach peak health.

24-29: You are doing some things well but could make some changes for your own benefit.

18-23: You have some major changes that need to be made.

12-17: Your health habits are not good. You need to implement some strategies to improve them.

Did you know?

Being aware of the areas that you need to improve is the first step to bettering your health. You must first admit you need to make the necessary changes and then take responsibility for improving them.

Wellness

WHEN YOU THINK of health, what comes to your mind? What are some signs that a person has bad health? What are some signs that a person has excellent health? How do we know if our health is improving or getting worse?

These are all excellent questions. Below are some of the common beliefs that people have regarding excellent health.

- ❖ Excellent health is about being thin.
- ❖ It means exercising a lot.
- ❖ It means avoiding foods that are bad for you.
- ❖ It means being able to conquer many tasks at once.

❖ It means having lots of friends and being happy all the time.

❖ It means being able to run a race fast.

❖ It is about not being sick.

The above thoughts come from a variety of sources, such as the media, common belief, and just an overall poor understanding of what health or, better yet, what wellness is. While nothing on that list is necessarily a bad thing, they are certainly not necessary for excellent health. There is no single thing or set of things that defines excellent health.

The old-school belief was that health is about not being sick. While not being sick is nice, today we have come to realize there is a lot more that goes into health. Excellent health is attained through a concept called wellness. As I like to say, everything is all about wellness!

Wellness is the balance between your physical, social, and mental health. The health triangle is made up of these three things—your physical, social, and mental health—kept in balance. Essentially, to achieve a high level of wellness, you need to be strong in each area and balanced.

The five essentials provide you with a blueprint on how to do well in the physical and mental sides. This book also has a full chapter geared toward the social side and how to keep strong relationships with a wide variety of people.

Below is a brief outline of what goes into each side of the wellness triangle.

Physical

- ✓ Are you maintaining a healthy weight?
- ✓ Are your measurements in the healthy range (e.g., blood pressure, cholesterol, etc.)?
- ✓ What is your resting heart rate?
- ✓ How often do you get viral or bacterial infections?

Mental

- ✓ Do you get angered easily?

- ✓ How well do you control stress?
- ✓ Do you believe you can complete challenges?
- ✓ Are you willing to take on new tasks?

Social

- ✓ Do you get along well with others?
- ✓ Do you have people to go to for advice?
- ✓ Do you have relationships with a wide variety of people?
- ✓ Are you able to listen and understand other points of view?

It is important to understand that each side of the health triangle connects to both other sides. For example, managing stress is important for your physical, social, and mental health. As you will find out, stress affects your body and mind. Stress can also affect the way you treat and communicate with others.

Besides this, we must understand that our wellness and our health are always changing. Have you ever suffered from an injury? Think about how that injury affected your mental health. Think about how that injury affected your social health.

We must understand that our health is never stable and is always changing. By following the five essentials, becoming health literate, and focusing on wellness, we can seek to improve every day.

Did you know?

Prior to the 1950s, good health was seen as simply the absence of disease. The term "wellness" was introduced in the United States in the 1950s by Halbert L. Dunn, M.D. He believed having a high level of wellness was integral to optimal body functioning.

Innate Intelligence

"YOUR BODY IS the best thing you ever got for free," said one of my health professors in college.

This is a very true statement! Your body is an amazing machine. When the body works the way it is supposed to and functions optimally, it is amazing. But when you are young, you may take your body and all its organs for granted.

As great as the body is, if you do not treat it right, it can lose its ability to heal and keep you healthy. You see, your body has an innate ability to want to heal itself and keep you at what scientists likes to call homeostasis, the point at which your body functions best. I like to refer to this as your body's innate intelligence. Basically, your body has the intelligence to heal itself automatically, without the help of medications or outside assistance, if everything is functioning optimally.

Think about it for a second. Have you ever gotten a cut or bruise? Did your body eventually heal and repair the damaged tissue? Have you ever gotten a cold or viral infection? Did your body heal from that and restore your health? The truth is the body can heal itself on the inside and outside. If we are healthy, we enhance our body's ability to do just that. On the other hand, if you make poor health decisions, your body's ability to heal itself can decrease over time.

Did you know?

Dr. Max Gerson (1881-1959) was a German physician who believed the body had an ability to heal itself from pretty much any disease. His belief was that all disease originates from lack of nutrients and high toxicity.

He developed an approach that involved eliminating toxins, drinking fresh juices, and consuming vegetarian foods to successfully treat patients with advanced diseases including cancer. Today, his approach is practiced at a clinic in Mexico that is run by his daughter, Charlotte Gerson.

(Sad Note: Unfortunately, Charlotte passed away at the age of ninety-six, during the publishing of this book.)

Why Be Healthy

WHEN THE DALAI LAMA was asked what surprised him most about humanity, he replied, "Man. Because he sacrifices his health in order to make money. Then he sacrifices money to recuperate his health."

This is true on so many levels. Many Americans are so focused on making money and enjoying pleasures that they neglect their health. Of course, this comes back to bite them in so many ways, through pain, sickness, loss of quality of life, and then their spending lots of money on medications.

If we want to get true enjoyment out of life, we need our health to be strong. There are countless benefits to having great health. The following are some of the benefits to being healthy:

- ❖ Having more energy and stamina
- ❖ Better focus and mental alertness
- ❖ Better muscle tone and a feeling of confidence
- ❖ Better performance in school or work
- ❖ Need for less medications, which means you save money
- ❖ Less stress and more enjoyment of life
- ❖ Higher life expectancy
- ❖ Stronger immune system, resulting in less illness
- ❖ Better relationships with family and friends
- ❖ Less anger and more happiness

Besides the list above, there are many other great benefits to having excellent health.

Your health should be at the top of your priority list. Without your health, life is very difficult. It is very hard to be a good parent, student, family member, co-worker, mentor, or role model without your health.

Don't ever feel you are being selfish for looking out after your health. Remember: when you are healthy and happy, then everyone around you will be happier, too.

###

Did you know?

The leading cause of bankruptcy in the United States is medical expenses.

Nutrition Basics

DO YOU EAT A variety of fruits and vegetables each day? Do you limit the amount of processed foods you eat?

The foods we choose to eat play a major role in our health. After all, nutrition is one of the essentials to health; you must put the right fuel in your body, if you expect it to perform well. In this brief section, we will discuss the basics of nutrition, and then later, we will discuss the science of nutrition in more detail.

There are six nutrients we get from food. Each of the nutrients plays a major role in our body's functioning. These six major nutrients are:

1. Carbohydrates
2. Proteins

3. Fats

4. Minerals

5. Vitamins

6. Water

The first three nutrients are considered the macronutrients. They provide the body with calories, which are the energy found in food. You can think of a calorie as a unit of energy that helps supply your body with the fuel it needs to function. Calories for your body are like gasoline for your car. Active people require more calories to function and recover from their workouts. We want to make sure we get calories from good sources of food that also supply our body with key nutrients.

Carbohydrates are a major energy source of the body; they break down into glucose and supply each cell with energy. Good sources of carbohydrates include fruit, vegetables, and whole grains.

In addition to carbohydrates, fats are also a major energy source in the body. Healthy fats include a wide variety of nuts, seeds, and fish. We should seek to consume healthy fats on a regular basis.

Proteins convert into amino acids, which are the building blocks of your cells and tissues. Great sources of protein are fish, lean meats, nuts, and beans.

One of the most basic concepts of nutrition is that the closer a food is to its natural state, the healthier it is for us. For example, fruits and vegetables are loaded with micronutrients (vitamins and minerals). But when they are processed, they lose a lot of their nutrients; then, other things that are not so good for us are added into it. Because of this, we should aim to make half of our plate at all meals should be made up of raw fruits and vegetables.

One important term to understand in nutrition is the term **nutrient density**. This refers to the amount of minerals and vitamins in a food compared to the number of calories. Foods that are low in calories but high in nutrients are considered very nutrient dense. On the other hand, foods that are low in nutrients but high in calories have low nutrient density. The most nutrient dense foods are plant foods. The following are good nutrient dense foods to consume everyday:

- ➢ Dark green vegetables (kale, spinach, and broccoli)
- ➢ Vegetables
- ➢ Fruits (berries, apples, and other fruits)
- ➢ Nuts and seeds
- ➢ Whole grains

When it comes to plant foods, we should eat a wide variety of colors. Different colors provide the different key vitamins and minerals our body needs to function. These vitamins and minerals do everything from keep our immune system strong to help our cells repair. In general, we should aim for lots of servings of fruits and vegetables each day.

Another great aspect of plant foods is that they are loaded with a nutrient called fiber. This is an essential nutrient that helps our food digest, keeps us feeling full, and can prevent cancers. Fiber is only found in plant foods—it's not found in non-plant foods—and it's very limited in processed foods. Our digestive system is happiest when we eat foods that are high in fiber.

Water is also very important! Most of our body consists of water, and without it, our body will not function well. Water does everything from keep your cells hydrated, help your brain function, and maintain your body temperature at homeostasis. In general, you should drink half your body weight in ounces each day. For example, a 160-pound person should aim for 80 ounces of water each day. If you exercise or are very active, then you should aim for even more water.

We should seek to limit or eliminate heavily processed foods and fatty meats. Not only are these foods low in key nutrients, but they also have bad chemicals added that are not good for us. The following types of foods should be limited or eliminated from our daily diets:

- ✓ Fast food
- ✓ Soda

- ✓ Baked goods (pastries, cakes, donuts, etc.)
- ✓ Candy
- ✓ Fatty meats

Did you know?

Plant-based foods have protein, too! We tend to think of protein foods as being meat, dairy, and eggs only. The truth is all plant foods have protein, and you can indeed get all your necessary proteins by consuming a wide variety of fruits, vegetables, and beans.

"The doctor of the future will no longer treat the human frame with drugs, but rather will cure and prevent disease with nutrition."

—Thomas Edison, 1908

Link Between Nutrition and Overall Health

THE FOODS WE consume not only affect our physical health but also our overall health. There is a strong link between the foods we consume and our performance in life in general.

Today, we see many kids diagnosed with ADHD, obesity, and diabetes. Without a doubt, this is affecting our kids' performance in many areas. We should seek to improve our diets, not only to maintain a healthier weight, but also so we increase our health and longevity.

As Charlotte Gerson states, our bodies have a natural healing mechanism, and we must nourish our bodies with the right balance of nutrients to function to our full potential.

In the developed nations, obesity is a major contributor to disease. Industry tells us obesity is the result of consuming too many calories, but the problem is much deeper than that. Contrary to popular belief, obesity is actually a sign of consuming too many low-nutrient-dense foods, according to Dr. Colin Campbell, author of the *China Study.*

All the processed foods we consume are depleted of nutrients because they are no longer in their whole form. Not only that, but most processed foods are low in fiber and do not fill us up, making it easy to over-eat. So, we eat more processed food, which gives us calories but does not fill the nutrient gap we are missing.

The key to beating obesity is not to focus on calories, like industry has us believing, but to eat a wide range of whole foods in their most natural state. These foods contain fiber, which keeps us feeling full and satisfied, and they give us a wide range of nutrients.

###

Did you know?

The book *Spark* by Dr. John Ratey discusses the amazing benefits of physical activity on the brain. Ratey shows that exercise provides many mental benefits, including focus and memory after exercise.

Organic Food

ACCORDING TO MICHAEL POLLAN, author of *The Omnivore's Dilemma,* organic food has many benefits over conventional. By definition, organic food is free from pesticides, sprays, and other chemicals. This is a big plus, because then our bodies just get the nutrients, vitamins, and enzymes from the plant and not any added chemicals.

Not only this, but, according to Pollan, organic food also has a wider variety of nutrients and vitamins due to the fact that it is grown in soil that is enriched with a wider variety of nutrients.

Organic food is also free of genetically modified crops, if you are concerned with that.

###

Did you know?

Some of the most heavily sprayed produce include apples, peaches, strawberries, grapes, cherries, nectarines, pears, and raspberries. Buying these organic will save you from pesticides and chemicals.

Natural versus Man-Made

IN GENERAL, the closer a food is to its natural state, the healthier it is for us.

When food is processed, excess sugar and fat are usually added, along with other bad chemicals oftentimes. Not only this, but processing food also damages and takes away many of the healthy nutrients that were originally in the food.

That does not mean we cannot enjoy an occasional treat every now and then, but, for optimal health, the vast majority of our diet should be clean and natural foods.

###

Did you know?

Unfortunately, today's soil is so depleted of key nutrients that our produce now lacks the same nutritional value it had fifty years ago. (Sorry for the bad news! I'll try to keep rest of these positive.)

Power of Plant Foods:

The Synergistic Effect

PLANT FOOD HAVE amazing benefits over processed food. As a rule of thumb, we should limit processed foods and animal proteins (meat, eggs, and dairy). That is, we should consume primarily vegetables, fruits, legumes, and whole grains.

Further, we should consume a wide variety of plant-based foods to ensure we get all the essential vitamins, minerals, and enzymes our body needs to function as a whole. I always tell people to think in terms of color. So, try to eat a wide variety of colors, including the dark green, red, and orange vegetables. (I know I continue to repeat myself about this. As they say, if the professor repeats it, then it must be important!)

The benefit of consuming plant-based foods is they have a relatively low glycemic index in comparison to processed foods. They also have lots of fiber and are more efficiently stored by the muscles and liver as energy, compared to high-sugar processed foods.

Colin Campbell conducted a study called the China Study that concluded humans eating mostly plant-based foods have fewer diseases, such as heart disease and cancer. Campbell concluded this was primarily due to the synergistic effect that occurs in the body when we eat a wide variety of plant-based foods.

Basically, all the vitamins and enzymes in plant-based foods work together to keep us healthy in a way no doctor or nutritionist could ever explain. Each vitamin, mineral, and enzyme in plant-based foods has an effect on the others that allows the entire body to remain healthy in a synergistic way.

Not only that, but plant-based foods also are loaded with antioxidants that help fight free-radical damage, again, and disease. As a rule of thumb, everyone should eat a wide variety of mostly plant-based foods, such as fruit and vegetables. For more information on nutrition, see the documentary *Forks over Knives*, which does a full overview of Campbell's China Study.

One of the effects of capitalism is that industry will always use its own criticism to its advantage. We see this a lot in the food industry! For example, "low fat," "low carbohydrates," "high in omega 3s," and the newest, "no high-fructose corn syrup."

Did you know?

In his book *The China Study*, Colin Campbell argues, if one consumes a plant-based diet, there is no need to worry about targeting specific nutrients. The reason is you will get the synergistic effect of the many nutrients and enzymes that are in plant-based foods.

Proteins

PROTEINS ARE AN important nutrient because they help to repair damaged muscle tissue. They also contain amino acids, which are the major building blocks of cells.

It is important to understand that all plant-based foods have some protein, and, if you eat a wide variety of plant-based foods, you can meet all your protein needs. That is not to say you have to be vegetarian for optimal health (for all you paleolithic and ketogenic folks out there).

The following are some excellent sources of proteins:

✓ Nuts, seeds, and beans

- ✓ Lean meats (chicken and turkey)
- ✓ Wild salmon
- ✓ Black bean burgers
- ✓ Greek yogurt

###

Did you know?

If you are exercising for longer than one hour, it is a good idea to consume a sports drink to replace key minerals lost. Nature's perfect sports drink is coconut water, as it has a mineral balance similar to human blood.

Carbohydrates

CARBOHYDRATES ARE your primary source of fuel (unless you are on the ketogenic diet). An important nutritional concept to understand is that all carbohydrates turn into sugar, which is utilized by your muscles and cells for energy. Your body breaks down stored sugar in your muscles and liver, known as glycogen.

Foods that serve as the best carbohydrate energy sources for the body are whole foods with plenty of fiber in them. Fruits, vegetables, and whole grains are your best sources of fuel, as they are easy on the digestive system and can be stored in your muscles and liver to be utilized as long-term energy.

Good choices include all fruits and vegetables, whole grain cereal, rice, pasta, and bread. When you are finished with a workout, you want to replace lost carbohydrates with simple sugars that immediately enter the blood stream. Great choices of post-workout foods include fruit juice and fresh berry smoothies.

###

Did you know?

The "low fat" craze of the 1980s was a large mistake and led to people being misinformed and encouraged to eat more high-sugar foods. These high-sugar foods are indeed low in fat, but eating them leads to obesity, when the body stores the extra sugar it doesn't use as fat.

Fats

HEALTHY FATS CAN be excellent sources of energy. Besides that, they can be great for your health, as they have good cholesterol, which can improve your overall health.

In general, excellent protein sources are also excellent sources of fat. The following are all good sources of fat:

- ✓ Almonds and cashews
- ✓ Other nuts and seeds
- ✓ Wild salmon
- ✓ Avocados
- ✓ Greek yogurt

###

Did you know?

The worst kind of fat are the transfats, which are labeled as partially hydrogenated oil on food labels. They became popular after saturated fats were identified as contributors to heart disease in the 1950s. Transfats are used in baked goods, snack foods, and margarine.

Vitamins and Minerals

YOUR MOTHER WAS right! We need to consume lots of fruits and vegetables.

Vitamins and minerals allow cellular repair and can prevent damage to the cells. To do this, we need to consume lots of nutrient-rich foods. Plant-based foods are very nutrient rich and contain lots of vitamins and minerals that will help your body repair.

One way to flood your body with lots of vitamins and minerals is to drink vegetable smoothies or fresh-pressed juice. The nutrients will be absorbed into your bloodstream more quickly from juices than smoothies, but both are a great way to load up on lots of micronutrients. Green juice or berry juice makes excellent nutrient-dense breakfasts; you can throw in some flax seeds for extra protein and omega-3 fatty acids.

It is extra important to consume a wide variety of fruits and vegetables during the day. The advantage to eating fruits and vegetables in their whole form is that you get the fiber, which keeps you full longer and slows down the sugar absorption in the body.

###

Did you know?

Juicing can be a great way to rebalance your body's nutrients. The best way to do this is to purchase a juicer and organic fruits and vegetables to juice on your own. Look up some great recipes.

"One-fourth of what you eat keeps you alive. Three-fourths of what you eat keeps your doctor alive."

—Dr. Andrew Saul

Processed Foods

AT THIS POINT, you are probably sick of hearing me say you should limit processed foods and consume more plant-based foods. Another concern with processed foods is the added chemicals and preservatives.

The truth is many of the chemicals put into processed foods in the United States are banned in other countries. For example, the European Union prohibits many food additives that are widely used in American foods.

Because industry has brainwashed consumers into thinking nutrition is all about calories, diet drinks have become very popular in our culture. The artificial sweeteners found in diet drinks and low-calorie foods are not healthy. Artificial sweeteners may trick the digestive system into thinking it is getting real sugar and consequently cause consumers of diet beverages to crave refined grains (hence, junk food) long term. Not only this, but these artificial sweeteners can have some bad side effects. Diet beverages are *not* a health drink. They can lead to weight gain and have serious side effects.

Next, food coloring dyes are not good, either. These dyes do nothing to enhance the nutritional value or taste of the food; they simply make the food look more appealing. They go under code names such as "yellow 5" or "blue 6," which means a mixture of other chemicals. Some of these food dyes have been banned in Europe due to various concerns the European Union had with them.

###

Did you know?

Do your research, read labels, and try to find quality products that do not use food dyes and artificial sweeteners. For example, stevia is a great low-calorie sweetener. Also, beta-carotene can be used instead of orange food dye.

Supplements

AS HUMAN BEINGS, it is critical we get all the vitamins, minerals, and enzymes we need in the right amount. This is why we want to consume foods in their natural whole form and not eat processed foods that have been depleted of nutrients. (I know: I said it again!)

Vitamins, minerals, and enzymes play a key role in keeping our bodies healthy and allowing our bodies to recover from the stress of life. The following is a list of nutrients that everyone should consider for optimal health and recovery. Of course, discuss these supplements with your health care provider first.

> ➤ **Vitamin D.** Vitamin D is also known as the sunshine vitamin. It is actually more of a

hormone than a vitamin. It regulates thousands of different functions in the body. Many studies support that high levels of vitamin D in the blood are effective in preventing diseases, including cancer.

➢ **Probiotics.** The human digestive tract has good bacteria that help food get absorbed and digested.

➢ **Omega-3s.** Current research supports that most Americans are too low in omega-3 fatty acids and too high in omega-6 fatty acids. It is optimal for us to have a ratio closer to three omega-6s to one omega-3; the ratio for most Americans is around 15 to 1. Good sources of omega-3s include flax seed, fish oil, and coconut oil.

➢ **Plant nutrients**. Consuming a variety of brightly colored fruits and vegetables is essential for optimal health and recovery. I prefer a product called Juice Plus.

###

Did you know?

Most people who live areas where there is a cold winter are low in vitamin D. Being low in vitamin D is not good for your immune system.

Calories

THE OBESITY EPIDEMIC in America is caused by people consuming more calories than their body burns. The energy balance equation states, if a person consumes more calories than their body burns, they will gain weight. If they burn off more calories than they consume, they will lose weight. Finally, if they consume the same amount as they burn, they will maintain their weight.

Even the most conservative dietitian would agree it is typically safe to consume 250 calories less than your body burns, if you are trying to lose weight. The problem begins when an individual cuts calories too much. Drastically cutting calories can lead to eating disorders and other health problems.

The average human burns around 2,500 calories per day, but an individual also burns calories in addition to this when they exercise. For example, a 150-pound runner burns roughly 150 calories per one-mile run. Cross-training and strength training activities burn calories, too, and should be factored into the caloric needs.

It is my opinion that an individual should turn the focus away from calorie-counting and look instead to consuming more nutrient-dense foods. Consuming lots of whole, plant-based foods such as fruits and vegetables are an easy way to make sure you do not overeat. In addition, plant-based foods have lots of fiber, which makes a person feel full and helps the nutrients digest easier.

I tell people their goal should be to consume ten different servings of organic fruits and vegetables every day. My belief is, if people focus more on the *quality* of foods they consume and less on the *calories*, they will be more successful with their weight-loss goals.

###

Did you know?

Even though I do not advise counting calories, it is a good idea to know how many calories your body burns per day. There are plenty of online calculators that can help you with that.

Popular Diets

ULTIMATELY, THE DEFINITION of "diet" is what a living organism consumes for survival. In other words, everyone is on a diet, even if you eat junk food all day long.

There is a lot of debate amongst the experts over the best way to eat for maximum health benefits. For example, Dr. Colin Campbell believes humans should consume a raw-food, plant-based diet, and Dr. Loren Cordain believes humans should eat a higher meat diet. Below is a summary of some of the common diets.

Paleolithic diet: The emphasis is on eating naturally raised meats, green vegetables, and other vegetables. The diet does not allow dairy products or grains. The idea is to eat like humans did during the Paleolithic era. This diet was created by Dr. Loren Cordain.

Mediterranean diet: This diet includes fish, dark greens, some fruit including olives and their oil, and whole grains. If dairy is consumed, it should be Greek yogurt. It also allows for red wine, dark chocolate, and feta cheese.

MyPlate: Diet promoted by the USDA. Includes a protein, vegetable, fruit, grain, and dairy product. Encourages eating a wide variety of foods.

Ketogenic diet: This is the ultimate low-carbohydrate diet. It encourages consuming a high proportion of protein and healthy fats. Its goal is to starve the body of carbohydrates and force the body to burn fat as fuel.

Vegan diet: This diet consists of only plant-based foods. In order to get all your nutrition needs, eating a wide variety of plant-based foods is important. This diet is emphasized by Dr. Colin Campbell in his book *The China Study.*

###

Did you know?

The Mediterranean diet was ranked as the best diet to prevent heart disease.

85

"Exercise is the best medicine. It just takes thirty minutes to swallow. Most importantly, it is free."

—Author unknown

Exercise Basics

DO YOU GET IN at least thirty minutes of physical activity every day? Are you able to go up a flight of stairs without losing your breath?

A college professor of mine told me, "Exercise is one of the best pills, and it just takes thirty minutes to swallow." This is true in so many ways! Regular physical activity is one of the best things we can do for our health and wellbeing. Not only does exercise improve your physical health, but it also enhances your mental health, too.

The benefits of exercise are endless. Regular physical activity will reduce your risk of pretty much every disease and improve your mental health. Below is a list of some of the many benefits to regular physical activity:

* Maintains a healthy weight and improves your muscle composition
* Lowers your blood sugar (high blood sugar is a major cause of disease)
* Reduces blood pressure and cholesterol levels in the body
* Lowers your resting heart rate, putting less stress on your heart
* Improves your lungs' ability to deliver oxygen to your body
* Improves bone density and reduces risk of osteoporosis
* Improves your immune system's ability to fight disease
* Improves overall stamina and energy
* Improves mood and reduces risk of depression
* Improves overall focus and memory
* Activates regions of your brain used in logical thinking

★ Can be done with friends and family as a way to strengthen relationships

We should do whatever exercise we enjoy and can maintain regularly. It is always a good idea to vary the activity and work different muscle groups. If you enjoy an activity, you are more likely to perform that exercise on a regular basis. Exercise should never seem like punishment, and if it does, you should seek out alternative activities you enjoy and can maintain.

The time you choose to exercise is up to you, and there are advantages to exercising at different times of the day. For example, morning exercise sessions can cause you to be more alert and energized the rest of the day. At the same time, you are more likely to pull a muscle in the early morning, so active stretching becomes very important.

A midday exercise session can be a great way to take a break away from the morning stresses. Your heart and muscles are strongest in the late afternoon, so you can often get better quality workouts at that time.

The old belief was that late-evening exercise negatively impacts sleep, but now current research says otherwise. Basically, we should exercise whenever it fits best in our schedule and we feel we can get the greatest benefit from the workout.

The bottom line is everyone should exercise regularly. What may differ between people, depending on their health, is the intensity of the exercise. Also, people who have bone and joint issues may seek exercises that have less impact, such as swimming or cycling. People should perform exercise that challenges them and can help improve their overall fitness. Of course, it is important to consult your doctor before starting any exercise program.

Did you know?

If you are feeling blue, try exercise as a cure. Research has shown that exercise can be effective in relieving mild to moderate depression. Exercise releases brain chemicals called endorphins that cause relaxation and a feeling of pleasure.

Stress/Recover/Adapt

WHEN YOU WORK OUT, your body believes you are working out for survival. For all your body knows, you are running away from a tiger or lifting a heavy rock to protect your life. Because of that, your body adapts to the stress and prepares itself better for the next fitness endeavor.

Your body is very smart and adapts to the stress put on it. Progression is a key principal to improving fitness. Fitness improves when the body is challenged. If the body is challenged too much, injury can result. The goal is, basically, to push your body slightly past its comfort zone and then recover, so your body can adapt to its new level.

Thus, it is very important for any person to slowly build on their level of fitness. It is also critical that everyone allow their bodies time to recover.

Did you know?

The body gets stronger after it has fully recovered from a workout. Take time to fully recover!

Body's Response to Exercise

WHEN YOU EXERCISE, all of the body systems are stressed in some way. All of the body systems must recover and be restored back to full health. This is why good nutrition, adequate water intake, sleep, stretching, and all the others parts essential for optimal recovery are critical. The idea is we train, stress the body systems out, and then let all the body systems return to full strength.

The human body is very smart, as it has a built-in healing mechanism that allows the body to recover completely from disease and breakdown. For example, if you cut yourself, the body eventually heals and recovers. And if you catch the flu, your body eventually defeats the virus and you are restored back to full strength.

When you stress your body through rigorous training and allow your body complete recovery, the body eventually recovers. Not only that, but your body bounces back even stronger than it was prior to the rigorous workout. This is the innate intelligence of your body at work, as it realizes it needs to better prepare itself for the next challenge.

Did you know?

The last system to recover from intense exercise is the nervous system. This is because the nervous system controls all of the other body systems including the immune system.

Building Fitness

IT IS IMPORTANT to understand the idea of stress, recovery, and adaption. The general idea is we stress our bodies by completing a workout, then we recover from that workout, and our body adapts to that level of fitness.

Let's say, for example, a couch potato begins to walk for thirty minutes and completes this workout five times each week. Since the couch potato went from no exercise to exercising regularly, she is going to see huge fitness gains within a few weeks. Then, after the fitness gains, if she does not work out any harder, she is not going to see any more improvements. She is just going to be able to maintain her current fitness.

I know lots of people who just continue to do what they have always done and never see any improvement, as a result. If we want to improve, we must increase the stress on our bodies progressively.

Our bodies get stronger during the recovery phase. That means, when we work out, we do not reap the benefits of that workout until our body is fully recovered, which is why it is important to take time and let the body recover after a workout.

After the body is done recovering, you will have reached a new level of fitness. You then have a window of time to complete another intense workout and increase fitness even more.

The key factor is to make the next intense workout more intense than the previous one. This can be done in the following ways:

- ➢ Shortening the recovery times, if doing intervals or repetitions.
- ➢ Lift more weight than you previously did before.

- ➢ Lift the same amount of weight, but do more repetitions.
- ➢ Simply go a longer distance or distances during repetitions.
- ➢ Attempt intervals at a faster pace for the same amount of time or distance.

Did you know?

It can take time to build fitness, so it should not be rushed into. Progression needs to be slow, and proper recovery time must be implemented.

High Intensity Interval Training (HIIT)

AS PART OF YOUR regular workout routine, you should periodically do High-Intensity Interval Training or HIIT. This is when you alternate between intervals of intense exercise followed by recovery. You can do HIIT with many modes of exercise, such as cycling, swimming, jump rope, squats, or running.

When doing high-intensity interval training, the recovery time, interval intensity, and interval length all factor into the stress of your workout. I recommend doing an active recovery, where you are at least walking during the recovery interval.

Some of the benefits of HIIT include stronger cardiorespiratory fitness, lower blood sugar, improved concentration after workouts, and release of mood-enhancing endorphins.

Some examples of great High Intensity Interval Training workouts are below:

- ☐ Pedal a stationary bike easy for ten minutes. Then pedal as fast as you can for thirty seconds followed by a one-minute easy pedal recovery. (Repeat ten times.). Cool down with five minutes of easy pedaling.
- ☐ Walk easy for five minutes. Then jump rope at an intense pace for forty-five seconds, followed by one minute of marching in place. (Repeat six times.) Then walk easy for five minutes.
- ☐ Run easy for eight minutes. Then run all-out for thirty seconds, followed by a one-minute active recovery. (Repeat ten times.). Bike easy for ten minutes.

The idea is you want to start with an easy warm-up, then do the fast intervals, and finish with an easy cool down. You can progressively increase the durations of your intervals, shorten recovery time, or do more intervals. Typically, you want to do HIIT about one to two times per week, depending upon fitness level.

###

Did you know?

The 7-minute Scientific Workout is a HIIT workout that engages the full body. The exercises are simple and can be done in seven minutes. Look it up!

Strength Training

STRENGTH TRAINING is a great addition to any exercise program. You can strength train with or without weights.

I recommend beginners strength train with their own body weight until they become more advanced. Once weights are involved, start with less weight and more repetitions. Make sure to pay attention to form and posture and safety recommendations.

Below is a possible strength training workout that you can do involving your own body weight. Start with the beginning stage for each exercise, and work your way to the next stage once you feel ready.

###

Exercise	Stage 1	Stage 2	Stage 3
Front plank:	30 sec.	1 min.	2 min.
Side plank:	15 sec.	30 sec.	1 min.
Calf raises:	15 reps	30 reps	60 reps
Leg kicks:	15/leg	30/leg	60/leg
Wall sits:	30 sec.	1 min.	2 min.
Push-ups:	15 reps	30 reps	60 reps
Dips:	20 reps	40 reps	80 reps
Superman:	30 sec	1 min.	2 min.

###

Did you know?

If one wants to increase muscle mass, they must consume plenty of nutrient dense foods and complete regular strength training workouts.

Core Strength

THE CORE CONSISTS of your abdominal muscles, back muscles, the muscles around the buttocks, and the muscles around the hips. A strong core reduces risk of injury and improves posture. Not only this, but your core muscles also help stabilize the foundation of your skeletal system, which is your spine. Because of this, a strong core can result in a more balanced posture and reduced likelihood of injury.

It is beneficial for individuals to perform various core exercises regularly, to gain additional core strength. The following is an example of a complete core routine:

###

Front plank: The front plank is a great isometric exercise that engages all of the core muscles.

Side plank: The side plank is a great isometric exercise that engages the stubborn muscles on the sides of the body.

Reverse crunch: This is a great exercise that works the lower abdominal muscles. Work your way up to two minutes' worth of reversed crunches.

Bicycle crunch: This is a great exercise that works the upper abdominal muscles and oblique abdominal muscles. Work your way up to two minutes' worth of bicycle crunches.

Superman: This is a great isometric exercise that works the back and hip muscles. Work your way up to holding the superman pose for two minutes.

Weight training: Weight training is a great way to engage the core in a variety of ways. Just make sure to not overdo the weight and to allow proper recovery time between sessions.

Yoga: Yoga is a great exercise that forces your core to remain engaged throughout each pose. Yoga is a great supplement to an exercise program.

Core workout videos: There are a variety of ten-minute core workouts that engage your core muscles in a variety of ways. Search your local bookstore or fitness store for some workout videos.

###

Did you know?

Yoga has been found to not only improve core strength, but also stress reduction.

Slow/Easy Training

THERE ARE MANY great benefits to exercising slow and easy. Your body needs to recover on the days following a hard workout. On these recovery days, you can help your body recover by doing a longer, slower, and easier workout.

For example, a nice thirty-minute elliptical session at an easy pace can help your blood vessels flush out lactic acid. Also, your cardiovascular system becomes stronger as a result of longer, slower exercise. The best exercise routine utilizes HIIT with these longer, slower workouts. Consider the following fun and easy workouts:

- ✓ Twenty-minute easy swim (great recovery after weight training)
- ✓ A one-hour hike
- ✓ Forty-five-minute easy bike ride
- ✓ Twenty minutes easy on a rowing machine
- ✓ A twenty to thirty-minute jog through the park

###

Did you know?

If you are exercising indoors, consider using a variety of machines, to engage different muscle groups.

Fad Exercise Programs

ANY TYPE OF EXERCISE is going to be beneficial for overall wellness. That said, stay mindful about fad exercise programs that promise quick results. The old saying that nothing of quality comes quickly is very true.

There are many fad exercise programs out there. The problem with these programs is they promote themselves as "one size fits all."

When doing an exercise program, it is all about listening to your body, as everyone recovers from workouts at a different rate. Make sure to give your body adequate time to recover between workouts. Most of all, find an exercise routine that is fun, something that you can keep up the rest of your life.

###

Did you know?

The issue with doing a video workout program is that they often do not account for the difference in recovery time between different people. If you are following a video workout program, make sure your body is fully recovered before starting a new intense workout.

Flexibility

FLEXIBILITY IS VERY important for a number of reasons. A flexible individual is less likely to get injured, will have better posture, and will recover from workouts better. Because of this, it is important for all athletes and everyone, in general, to work on flexibility on a regular basis.

Flexibility can be improved through dynamic and static motion stretches. The key areas of flexibility are calves, hamstrings, quadriceps, hip flexors, and back. One of the best ways to improve flexibility in these areas is to practice yoga on a regular basis.

Learn a few basic yoga poses, and perform them for ten minutes at the end of a workout. Over time, you should see your flexibility improve. It is also a great idea to learn some basic static stretches and perform them at the end of a workout, too. I discuss some ideas and options in the next few sections.

Did you know?

Yoga is a great way to improve flexibility and mental health. Yoga classes are held at a variety of places, including health clubs.

Dynamic Stretching

DYNAMIC STRETCHING simply refers to stretches that involve movement of the targeted muscle. The goal is to gradually stretch the targeted muscle through movement.

Dynamic stretching is the type of stretching that should be done before every workout. Besides getting the muscle ready for activity, dynamic stretching also creates a better connection between your nervous system and muscles.

Examples of great dynamic stretches to do prior to a workout include:

➢ butt kicks
➢ high knees

> side steps

> lunges

> calf raises

> back twists

> jumping jacks

> arm circles

> leg swings

###

Did you know?

When on a road trip, consider stopping every hour or so and doing these dynamic stretches. They can prevent stiffness later on.

Static Stretching

STATIC STRETCHING is a great way to improve your range of motion. Increasing your range of motion will decrease your chance of injury and make you a faster runner.

The best time to static stretch is after your workout is complete. You want to make sure to hold each stretch for at least thirty seconds and progress into the stretch gently.

The science behind improving flexibility is the same as improving other areas of fitness. You must overload the muscle you are trying to stretch and progressively increase your range of motion. You should never stretch to the point of pain or severe discomfort, however.

Gentle static stretching is also a great way to help your body recover in the days following a challenging workout. Make sure to stretch out your calves, hamstrings, lower back, hip flexors, and quadriceps.

###

Did you know?

The best time to improve flexibility is following a workout, as your muscles are warm and will stretch best.

Foam Rolling

FOAM ROLLING is a great way to help boost the recovery of your muscular system and also enhance the performance of your nervous system during a workout.

Get yourself a large foam roller, and roll all of your lower-extremity muscles several times each week, post-workout. I believe in foam rolling prior to static stretching as a way to prepare large muscles for activity and enhance recovery.

Make sure to roll each of the major muscle groups of the legs—the hamstrings, calves, and quadriceps—as well as the lower back.

###

Did you know?

If you have never foamed rolled before, it may be quite painful at first, but, after a while, the muscles adapt.

Chiropractic Care

CHIROPRACTIC CARE is a great addition to your recovery program. Contrary to popular belief, chiropractors do a lot more than make your back feel better. Chiropractors adjust your spine, which is the foundation of your skeletal system.

Your spine runs all the way from the base of your brain to your tailbone. When the three curves of your spine are in the optimal positions, your skeletal system is better able to absorb the shock of movement, so you will be able to move with more efficiency and your overall body will be balanced, decreasing the chance of injury.

When it comes to chiropractors, they are all over the board on what they claim they can do. Find a chiropractor who understands fitness and is willing to listen to your concerns. A good chiropractor should examine your spine based on an x-ray, explain to you the results of your x-ray, and offer their plan on correcting problem areas.

A lot of world-class athletes see a chiropractor several times a week. I believe everyone would benefit from seeing a chiropractor regularly.

Just a fair warning, though: many of your friends will discourage you from visiting chiropractors. Chiropractors have gotten bad-mouthed over the years for being quacks and just wanting your money. Nothing could be further from the truth! They attempt to heal the skeletal system and human body using natural methods and without drugs. Many people who visit a chiropractor regularly find themselves feeling more energetic, getting sick less, and just feeling better overall.

###

Did you know?

The science behind chiropractic care is that the brain and spinal cord send messages throughout your whole body. Chiropractors work to relieve your spinal cord of interference, known as subluxations. By removing the subluxations, the belief is your body's nervous system is in the best position to heal itself.

Massage Therapy

MASSAGE THERAPY has its advantages when it comes to recovery and relaxation of muscles. A massage will get the blood and lymphatic fluid flowing through your body, allowing for better detoxification and recovery.

If you can afford it, a weekly massage is a great idea. You can also use foam rollers, massage rollers, and other tools to give yourself a massage. I personally use a foam roller and a running tool called "the Stick" almost every day pre- and post-workout.

Did you know?

Poor posture is the reason for a lot of muscle pain that people have. In particular, slouching and looking down at a cell phone can cause your neck muscles to become out of whack.

Pain Killers and Anti-Inflammatory Medications

UNFORTUNATELY, MANY people, including athletes, resort to medications to push through pain. This is a bad idea for many reasons.

There are lots of studies to support that regular use of anti-inflammatory and narcotic drugs increases the risk of injury and further damage to the body. Prescription narcotics block pain receptors that communicate to the body that something is wrong. At the same time, narcotics do nothing to help the body heal or improve health.

Furthermore, narcotic medications are very dangerous and can lead to addiction and liver damage.

It is my opinion that an athlete who relies on over-the-counter or prescription medication to get through workouts should take time off or back away from their training. I take a very strong stance against both narcotic pain killers and ant-inflammatory medications.

The following are excellent ways to improve recovery and promote healing that do not involve drugs:

> Chiropractic care
> Massage therapy
> Foam rolling
> Pain relief creams (Biofreeze, Icy Hot, etc.)
> Ice
> Heat

Did you know?

The pharmaceutical industry and medical field have largely been criticized for creating the opiate epidemic in America by pushing narcotic medications on patients.

"A good laugh and a long sleep are the two best cures for anything."

—Irish Proverb

Sleep

DO YOU WAKE UP fully energized every day? Do you feel like you need a midday nap at times? As you probably know, sleep is a vital component to health.

When you sleep at night, you go through sleep cycles. Each sleep cycle is about ninety minutes long; the final ten to twenty minutes of each cycle are vital. This component of the sleep cycle is called rapid eye movement (REM) sleep.

During REM sleep, your body and brain repair, muscles shut down, and memories are stored. Prior to REM sleep, your body also goes through various changes during sleep. The following are some of the changes that occur during a night's sleep:

- ✓ Heart rate lowers
- ✓ Breathing rate lowers
- ✓ Muscles relax and shut down during REM sleep
- ✓ Tissues and cells repair
- ✓ The immune system gets a boost
- ✓ Memories are converted from short to long term
- ✓ Growth happens during the pre-adult years

Not getting enough sleep at night will affect your next day in many ways. For starters, you won't be as focused, energetic, and alert. Sleep experts agree that the symptoms of sleep deprivation are close to that of the common attention deficient disorders. For example, inability to focus, poor memory, and lack of self-control are symptoms of sleep deprivation.

Also, one of the obvious symptoms of sleep deprivation is being easily angered, something that will affect your relationships with others. Since memories are converted from short-term to longer-term memory during sleep, your ability to learn and recall information will also be impacted.

Long-term sleep deprivation can be fatal. Your body needs the benefit of the recovery that happens when you get quality sleep; without it, your overall health will be impacted. When you deprive yourself of sleep, your immune system is weaker, increasing your risk of every disease. Sleep deprivation also negatively affects your brain, causing memory problems and increasing risk of depression. When you are younger, not getting enough quality sleep can affect growth and muscle development.

To prevent both the short- and long-term problems that occur with sleep deprivation, it is important for every person to get enough quality sleep each night. Quality sleep is just as important as the quantity of sleep that you get. The following tips will help you get the best quality sleep each night:

➢ Keep a consistent sleep schedule by trying to go to bed and wake up at the same time every night.

➢ Adults should aim for at least eight hours of sleep each night.

➢ Avoid caffeine after 2:00 pm as its stimulating effects can keep you awake at bedtime.

➢ Eat dinner at least three hours before your bedtime.

➢ Keep your room as dark as possible.

➢ Avoid having a television on right before bed; it's best not to have a television in your bedroom.

➢ Listen to soothing music or do some light reading before bed.

➢ Sleep on your side or back but not on your stomach (extended stomach-lying is bad for the spine and neck).

➢ Eat a piece of fruit before bed, and drink a glass of water or herbal tea.

➢ Make sure your mattress and your pillow are comfortable and support your back and neck.

➢ Keep your cell phone away from your bed, as it can be a distraction.

###

Did you know?

Have you ever woken up naturally but decided to go back to bed and wait for the alarm, only to find yourself super-tired when the alarm clock goes off? This is because your alarm clock woke you up in the middle of the sleep cycle. You will naturally wake up after a full sleep cycle, but if you get woken up in the middle of a sleep cycle, you will be extra-groggy.

Minimizing Toxins

WE BRIEFLY DISCUSSED the importance of good nutrition and putting good quality nutrients in your body. This includes mostly plant foods that provide your body with an array of vitamins and minerals.

The truth is, even if you are putting nutrient-dense foods in your body, you can ruin the benefit by taking in too many toxins. Toxins are chemicals that are foreign and unrecognizable to the body. Your body attempts to get rid of toxins and usually does a very good job of that, but sometimes they can become overbearing.

An easy example of that is the damage too much tobacco or alcohol will do to your body over time. To this day, smoking is the leading behavior that contributes to an early death. If we are going to take our health seriously, we must look for ways to reduce our exposure to toxins.

There are many ways we can be exposed to toxins daily. For example, the toxin in soda known as phosphoric acid can weaken teeth and bones. Secondhand smoke can be just as damaging as smoking directly. It is important to recognize the common ways we are exposed to toxins and then seek to reduce your exposure to them. The following is a list of some of the ways we are exposed to toxins:

- Preservatives and chemicals in processed food, including food dyes
- Caramel coloring, phosphoric acid, sodium benzoate, and other chemicals found in soda
- Excessive sugar in the form of high-fructose corn syrup found in processed foods
- Chemicals found in skin lotions, including sun screens

- Tobacco smoke, including secondhand smoke
- Chemicals inhaled through e-cigarettes (vapes)
- Alcohol
- Medications (prescription and over the counter)
- Illicit drugs
- Too much sunlight (cause of skin cancer)
- Too much caffeine
- Pollution
- Pesticides

We should seek to prevent as many toxins from getting in our bodies as we can. The following tips will help you avoid or eliminate exposure to many of the common toxins:

- Limit processed, packaged, and fast foods.
- Buy organic fruits and vegetables to avoid pesticides.

* Stay away from people who smoke, and avoid buildings with smokers.

* Limit or eliminate alcohol consumption.

* Do your research on sunscreens and skin lotions, and purchase those made with natural minerals.

* Ask your doctor if any natural treatment options are available. Try to avoid painkiller medications at all costs, and seek natural pain relief (e.g., icing, massage, heat, stretching, and chiropractic care).

Our body is very efficient at getting rid of toxins, if we treat it right. There are certain things we can do to help our body get rid of toxins. The following is a good list of healthy detox habits to get into:

* Drink plenty of water, as water can help dilute some of the pollution entering our bodies.

* Eat lots of dark-green organic vegetables, as they help your body get rid of toxins.

* Exercise as a means of sweating out more toxins.
* Spend some time in a steam room or sauna to help your body sweat.
* Eat as clean a diet as possible to avoid putting processed foods in your body.
* Consume a diet high in fiber by eating a lot of plant-based foods.

###

Did you know?

Many of the common toxins in processed food in the United States are banned in European countries.

Alcohol

ALCOHOL ABUSE continues to be a major problem in the developed world. For whatever reason, our society tends to look at alcohol as a friendly drug, and it is widely celebrated. Nothing can be further from the truth!

Alcohol is one of the most toxic drugs known to man, and it does not take long for alcohol to poison you. Alcohol is rapidly absorbed in your blood stream and brain within seconds of drinking it. It can affect your coordination, memory, emotions, decision making, and speech, along with your entire body's ability to function. Long-term alcohol use has been linked to liver damage and an increased risk for select cancers.

###

Did you know?

Alcohol is a depressant drug, which means it slows down your entire nervous system.

Smoking and Vaping

SMOKING CONTINUES to be the leading cause of chronic disease in the developed world today. The nicotine in tobacco is very addicting and makes it difficult for a smoker to quit smoking. While the smoker claims a cigarette relaxes them, it is just satisfying the addiction they have.

There are many toxic and carcinogenic chemicals in a cigarette, and because of that, smoking greatly increases your risk of heart disease and every type of cancer. Your best bet is to not start smoking.

Electronic cigarettes have become very popular amongst teenagers. Many users falsely believe that these e-cigarettes are safe. Electronic cigarettes contain nicotine, and because of that, users have an increased risk of becoming tobacco user.

There are also hundreds of chemicals in e-cigarettes, and these chemicals can cause lung damage. More information is needed on the long-term effects of these electronic cigarettes, but it is safe to assume they will be damaging in the long run.

###

Did you know?

Nicotine is one of the most addictive drugs known to man.

"Words are powerful. They have the
ability to create a moment and the strength
to destroy it."

—Susan Gale

Mental Health

WHEN YOU WAKE UP, are you excited for the challenges that lie ahead? The truth is most people wake up and immediately begin to think negative thoughts. That is, many people mentally beat themselves up before they even start their day. It is important for us not to do this!

Your actions are always a reflection of your thoughts. If you think more positive thoughts, you will get better results. In this section, I wish to analyze the way we think and the impact that thoughts can have on your health.

Most of the mental toxins we allow to enter our mind are thoughts related to fear, failure, anger, jealousy, greed, sadness, and anxiety. If we allow these mental toxins to fill our mind, then we will never get the most out of our life. These toxins not only cause us to think negatively, but they also prevent us from reaching our peak potential. It is important for us to remember that thoughts affect our physical health as well as our mental health. (Later on, we will discuss how stress affects your physical body in a negative way.)

One way to get rid of toxic thoughts is to simply fill your mind with nurturing thoughts. I like to think of these nurturing thoughts as vegetables for your mind. They help your mind detoxify, and they nourish it with positive energy. We simply function better when we are in a state of compassion and bliss.

The following are thoughts and actions that lead to a better overall health:

- Being happy for others
- Putting yourself in others' shoes, and having compassion
- Volunteering to help those in need
- Being grateful for what you do have

- ➤ Greeting change with excitement
- ➤ Being optimistic about your chances of success
- ➤ Taking on a growth mindset in new challenges

The following is a set of quotes that should help put your mindset in the right spot:

- ✳ "Make forgiveness your highest function; that means forgive others and yourself."
- ✳ "Greet change with openness and expect that change will happen."
- ✳ "Take time to ponder and meditate. Enjoying the present moment is key."
- ✳ "Let your dreams be your guide, not your fears"
- ✳ "True failure is the act of giving up"

###

Did you know?

The placebo effect has been shown to work multiple times. The simple belief that a person has an advantage is oftentimes enough to actually help them improve.

Controlling Stress

DO YOU FIND yourself stressed out all the time? Are you easily angered? Does life feel difficult most of the time? Do you feel you are unable to control your stress? If you answered yes to any of these questions, your stress may be taking a toll on your health.

Imagine you are enjoying a picnic on a nice sunny day. You are with your friends, enjoying fun games and good food. Then, out of nowhere, comes this large angry bear. The bear looks furious, and immediately you feel threatened. You now have a choice to either run away from the bear or fight the bear.

Imagine how the threat of the bear will change the physiology of your body. Your heart rate will go up, breathing will become faster, muscles will tense, blood pressure increases, blood sugar increases, sweating begins, your senses will sharpen, and your brain will switch into survival mode. These changes will help you either fight or run away from the bear. On the other hand, any body system not needed to run away or fight will turn off. This includes your digestive, reproductive, and immune systems.

In the bear example, it is beneficial for your body to go through the stress response. After all, the stress response will put you in the best position to run or fight the bear. For the most part, the stress response is only useful when our life is in immediate danger.

The problem is humans let themselves get in the stress response for things that are not life-threatening. Our adrenal glands store adrenaline for emergency response to a threatening situation. We do not want to tap into this adrenaline too often, or it can damage our body's ability to heal.

When it comes to your health, stress is not your friend. Because your immune system is shut off during the stress response, constant stress increases your risk of getting sick.

The following is a list of some of the short-term effects stress has on the body:

- ✓ Muscles get more tense
- ✓ Pupils dilate
- ✓ Sense of hearing improves
- ✓ Logical thinking is impaired, and reptile brain turns on
- ✓ Heart rate and breathing increase
- ✓ Blood pressure rises
- ✓ Blood sugar rises
- ✓ Immune system is impaired
- ✓ Digestive system is impaired
- ✓ Reproductive system is impaired

The short-term effects of stress are your body's response to get out of danger. The problem becomes when we are constantly under stress and our body's systems eventually become overloaded.

The following are some of the long-term effects of chronic stress:

- ✓ Higher risk of heart diseases (due to wear and tear on your heart and blood)
- ✓ Higher risk of viral and bacterial infections (due to immune system being decreased)
- ✓ Back aches and headaches (due to muscle tension)
- ✓ Digestive and reproductive system problems (due to impairment of these systems)
- ✓ Higher risk of depression
- ✓ Anger levels may get higher

Because of the dangerous short- and long-term effects of stress, it is important we manage our stress. Stress cannot be eliminated from our lives, but it can greatly be reduced by coming up with a good stress management action plan.

This action plan will look different for everyone. The following are some tips on managing stress.

> Make sure to get regular physical activity. The activity can be anything that you want, but make sure to exercise for at least thirty minutes daily.

> Make sure to get enough sleep. Sleep is critical to reducing stress! If you miss out on sleep, you will be under more stress in the short and long term.

> Learn relaxation exercises that can help your body get out of the stress response. Possible relaxation exercises are yoga, meditation, deep breathing, and guided imagery.

> Take time to do things you enjoy. As simple as this sounds, it is amazing how many people do not do this.

> For some, reading, art, or puzzles is a great way to manage stress.

> Avoid dangerous activities that many people use to deal with stress, such as alcohol, drugs, or violent behavior.

> ➢ Explore different stress-management techniques, and you should soon learn what works for you.

Did you know?

Stress can come from both external and internal sources. It can be argued most of the stress we experience today comes from our own thoughts. Because of this, you can reduce your stress by changing the way you think and by framing your thoughts in a different way.

Two great questions to ask yourself when you feel stress coming on are: Is my life in danger? Will the stress response help the situation? If the answer is no to both, then tell yourself that stressing out is not worth it.

Relaxation Exercises

CHANGING THE WAY you think and following a healthy lifestyle can greatly reduce the amount of stress in your daily life. Adequate sleep, nutrition, and exercise are three key areas to combat stress. In addition to these, I would like to introduce another lifestyle behavior that can greatly reduce your overall stress and improve your health: relaxation exercises. There are several relaxation exercises you can experiment with to see which ones work best for you. Like anything, it takes regular practice with them to get the benefits.

Each of these relaxation exercises are designed to get your body out of the stress response. When you get your body out of the stress response, your body is in the best position to heal itself.

The relaxation exercises below are very simple and can be done by anyone. You get the best benefit from these exercises when you do them regularly. There are others not mentioned in this book, but these are the ones I have had the greatest success with.

Meditation:

- Find a comfortable place free of distractions.
- Sit down, and keep your posture balanced. Do not slouch!
- Place your hands wherever you want.
- Decide on a word or phrase to repeat.
- Close your eyes, and continue to repeat the word or phrase in your mind
- Your only intention is to get back to that word. If your mind drifts away, just focus on repeating the word or phrase.
- Perform for about ten to twenty minutes.
- Come out of the meditation slowly!

Guided Imagery:

- Look up a guided-imagery video.

- You can sit or lie down on your back.
- Close your eyes and listen to video.
- Come out of the guided imagery exercise slowly.

Deep breathing:

- Take five deep breaths in and out.
- Ask yourself: *Is my life in danger?*
- Ask yourself: *Is being in the stress response helpful?*
- Your answer should always be *no* to both questions, unless you really are in danger.
- Then take five deep breaths again.

Did you know?

Studies show that meditation activates the deep brain waves that otherwise are only activated during deep sleep, promoting recovery.

"Everything you want is on the other side of fear."

—Jack Canfield

Conquering Fear

FEAR IS THE EMOTION that comes from the thought, *If I do this, then something bad will happen.* Fear is only useful in instances when it prevents us from doing something that may damage us. For example, fear is what prevents you from crossing the street when a car is coming. Fear is what prevents you from gambling away all your money at a casino. Fear is completely natural and useful in many instances.

The problem arises when we let fear stop us from growing as an individual. When you are afraid to take smart risks, you limit your capabilities as an individual. Because of this, we need be aware of the fears we have and be willing to conquer them.

For example, many people fear what others will think of them. This is common and something we do not want to fear. If we spend our whole life worrying about what others think of us, we will not accomplish much. Never let your wellness or personal growth suffer because of fear of what others may think of you.

The following are some tips on conquering your fears:

> Look up the statistics on your fear. For example, you have a better chance of being in a car accident than a plane accident.
> Realize that experience is key to getting over your fear. For example, the best way to conquer a fear of public speaking is to do it several times.
> Talk about your fear with someone who does the thing you're afraid of, and come up with strategies to overcome it
> Realize no fear is common among all people; there are always others who do not share your fear.

➢ Admit your fear and realize that it can be unlearned.

Did you know?

It has been said that more people fear public speaking than death. Once you free yourself of the fear of what others think, you become free as an individual to express yourself.

"He who angers you, controls you."

—Author unknown

Anger Management

MANAGING YOUR ANGER is critical for gaining control of your mental health. Anger comes from the thought, *This should not be happening right now*. Think about it! Every time you have gotten angry in the past, this thought always raged through your mind.

Like fear and stress, anger is given to us for survival reasons. About the only time anger does us any good is in situations where something or someone is attacking us. Then, anger causes our adrenaline to go up and puts us in the best position to fight the attacker.

When we let anger flood our mind, it really affects our health and thinking. We do not think well when we are in a state of anger. There is a lot of truth to the saying anger makes us stupid. For our health and relationships, it is essential we learn to manage our anger.

The following are tips for managing anger:

- Take stress-management seriously, and continue to manage your stress.
- Perform relaxation exercises such as meditation and yoga on a regular basis.
- Keep up with an exercise routine. Exercise enhances our mood!
- Reflect on why you got angry, and keep a journal.
- Make sure to get enough sleep, as sleep deprivation leads to getting angry quickly.
- Always try to respond in an assertive, kind, and compassionate manner.

###

Did you know?

One of the first signs of sleep deprivation is being easily angered.

"If you are searching for that one person that will change your life, take a look in the mirror."

—Author unknown

Visualization

VISUALIZING YOURSELF reaching your goals is an important part of the process. Many successful athletes use visualization as a tool to help them reach peak performance.

Billy Mills, who won the 10,000 metres gold medal at the 1968 Tokyo Olympics, visualized himself winning the race dozens of times every day for years before the race. Once race day came, he pulled off one of the greatest upsets in Olympic history.

I suggest creating a vision board for yourself and updating it regularly. Vision boards can be created on your smart phone, computer, or on paper. Put pictures of images that represent yourself reaching your goals and affirmations. Display it somewhere where you can see it regularly.

Visualization helps your mind perceive success before it happens. As Billy Mills says, the subconscious mind does not know the difference between reality and imagination.

Did you know?

Vision boards allow you to use imagery as a way to ignite your passion, goals, and affirmations. Making an electronic vision board is great because you can update it easily with your new goals.

Affirmations

SETTING AFFIRMATIONS is a great way to change behavior. An affirmation is a positive statement, usually written in "I am" form. Writing the affirmation down on paper, posting it in as many places as possible, and repeating it to yourself regularly are keys to the process.

You want to set affirmations toward areas of your life that you tend to think negatively about, which likely causes you not to perform well. For example, if you feel you do not make good dietary choices, you could set an affirmation toward healthier eating.

Your affirmation may be something along the lines of, "I eat healthy foods every day." By writing this down and repeating it to yourself, you should notice, after some time, your dietary choices will be better. For example, you may choose a piece of fruit instead of a candy bar as a snack. Over time, you should notice yourself making better choices around your nutrition.

When creating affirmations, it is important to state them in the present tense. Affirmations are not goals! They need to be written in the form that shows you presently have that skill or trait. Affirmations work at realigning thoughts in your mind so that, eventually, you repeat more positive thoughts.

It will take time and practice to successfully change your thoughts. You will find yourself swaying off of your affirmation every now and then. When this happens, it is important to continue to repeat the affirmation in your head and not give up. Continue to repeat it, and you will notice that positive changes will happen.

Did you know?

An effective affirmation works to "re-wire" your subconscious mind to spit out more positive thoughts in your conscious mind. It will take time to "re-wire" your subconscious mind.

Suicide Prevention

UNFORTUNATELY, SUICIDE continues to be a major problem. In fact, suicide is the third leading cause of death amongst people in the United States fifteen to twenty-four years of age, after car accidents and homicides.

The following are common warning signs of suicide:

- ☐ If a person talks about killing themselves or having no reason to live
- ☐ Increased use of drugs and alcohol
- ☐ Withdrawing from normal activities
- ☐ Isolating themselves from others
- ☐ Looking for ways to end their lives online

- ☐ Giving away prized possession
- ☐ Major mood changes
- ☐ Constant depression, anxiety, or irritability

The list above by no means includes all the possible warning signs.

Warning signs should not be ignored. You should encourage the person to get help as soon as possible. For any youth you suspect as suicidal, telling a trusted adult of his or hers is vital.

###

Did you know?

The National Suicide Prevention Hotline is 1-800-273-8255. It is available twenty-four hours per day, 365 days per year!

"If you do what you've always done,
you'll get what you've always gotten."

—Tony Robbins

Goal Setting

AFTER LEARNING ABOUT the five essentials to health, you probably have an idea of the essentials you are strong at and weak in.

For example, you may exercise regularly, but you know you could benefit by eating healthier. Or you may exercise and eat healthy, but you know you do not get enough quality sleep and are always stressed out.

One of the best ways to improve your overall wellness is to focus on the essentials you know need improvement and then to set goals. Goal-setting is a powerful technique that forces you to commit to improvement.

In this section, we are going to focus on a goal-setting technique called SMART goals. You may have heard of them before, as SMART goal-setting is used by many companies, schools, and sports teams all over the world.

The way you format your goal is very important. To give yourself the best chance of success, format your goal using the SMART goal-setting process, and write it down.

A good goal contains each part of the SMART goal-setting acronym. After you format your goal, make sure it contains each part below:

Specific: Your goal should be stated in a way that tells you exactly what you wish to accomplish.

Measurable: At the end of a designated period of time, you should be able to check off whether you met or did not meet your goal.

Attainable: Your goal should be something you can achieve and find worthwhile to achieve.

Realistic: Your goal should be a real possibility for you.

Time-bound: Your goal should have a deadline for when you will complete it by.

Remember: how you write and format your goals is very important. For example, most New Year's resolutions fail because they are not written as SMART goals. A good goal contains each element of the SMART goal-setting process. When your goal is written in this format, it is easier to assess your progress toward the goal. If your goal is missing an element, it is easier to fall off track.

Here are some bad examples of goals:

- ✓ I will eat healthier (not specific and not time-bound)
- ✓ I will run faster than five minutes in the mile (not time-bound)
- ✓ I will practice mediation regularly (not time-bound or specific enough)

✓ I will exercise daily (not specific in terms of how long)

Here are some good examples of goals:

* I will eat five servings of plant-based foods daily.
* I will exercise every day for at least twenty minutes.
* I will keep a journal of my daily relaxation activities.
* I will run the mile in seven minutes or faster by the end of the year.

It is important to set both long-term goals and short-term goals. You can create a goal-setting plan that consists of a long-term goal and then a few short-term goals. The short-term goals should be designed in a way that get you closer to reaching your long-term goal.

For example, your long-term goal may be to run the mile in eight minutes or faster by the end of the year. A short-term goal that would help would be to run for at least fifteen minutes, five times per week. Short-term goals help you focus on improving and make it easier to track performance.

It is important to understand the difference between process goals and outcome goals. Outcome goals focus on achieving a specific result. For example, a basketball team may set the goal of winning ten games in a season.

On the other hand, process goals focus on performing a behavior in a certain way or doing something a certain number of times. An example of this would be setting a goal to exercise twenty minutes per day. Both types of a goals are great, but setting process goals gives you more control over achievement of your goal. Often, outcome goals can be set and then process goals can be created to get closer to reaching your outcome goal. Here is an example below.

Outcome goal: I will lose ten pounds by the end of the year.

Process goal 1: I will exercise twenty minutes daily.

Process goal 2: I will eat at least five servings of fruits and vegetables daily.

Process goal 3: I will only have three caloric beverages per week.

Finally, all goals need to be monitored and adapted to circumstances over time. For example, if you set a goal to run a 5k in under twenty-two minutes but, on race day, it is twenty degrees and snowing with icy roads, you may need to change your goal.

It is much easier to stay focused on goals when they can measured frequently and are short-term goals. I am not saying that saying that all goals have to be short-term goals, but you may want to set some short-term sub-goals to go with your long-term goal.

###

Did you know?

Writing down your goals and displaying them greatly increases the chances you will follow through with your goals.

Maintaining a Healthy Weight

IT IS NO SECRET that obesity is a major problem in the United States and other developed countries. In fact, roughly two out of every three adults are considered overweight and, of those, about one out of every three is considered obese.

Obesity not only affects adults but is also beginning to affect children, as more and more kids are becoming obese. Obesity was not such a large problem decades ago, but it is getting even worse every day. As discussed earlier, obesity and tobacco smoking are the two leading contributors to all the major diseases that plague Americans today.

The following are some of the reasons for the obesity epidemic:

- The amount of physical jobs done by Americans has gone down; nowadays, more Americans are working less active jobs, due the increase of technology.

- The increase of video games and television programs has caused children and adults to entertain themselves without physical activity.

- Our food system has made poor-nutrient-dense foods really cheap, while healthy food remains expensive. (Read Michael Pollan's book, *The Omnivore's Dilemma,* for more information.)

- Americans' stressful "on the go" lifestyles have caused many to turn to fast food for quick, cheap meals.

When it comes to maintaining a healthy weight, it mainly comes down to exercise and nutrition habits. My chiropractor, Dr. Jasbir Kochar, likes to remind me that nutrition is king and exercise is queen.

The following are some helpful tips on ways to maintain a healthy weight:

* Focus on nutrient-dense foods. Nutrient-dense foods are mostly plant-based foods. Fruits and vegetables keep you full and make you less likely to overconsume on high-caloric foods. Make half your plate fruits and veggies!

* Exercise daily! Try and do a variety of physical activities, including weight lifting, to improve your muscle mass and increase your metabolism. Remember: any exercise is better than no exercise.

* Drink plenty of water! Drinking water causes your body to burn more calories.

* Avoid or greatly limit liquid calories, including alcohol, soda, and juices. These beverages are loaded with calories and will not keep you full.

* Take sleep seriously! Getting adequate sleep improves your metabolism and makes you crave less junk food.

* Control your stress! As part of the stress response, you are more likely to crave sugar.
* In general, portion control is more important than avoiding certain foods. Enjoy your favorite foods in moderation.
* Avoid fad diets, and aim for lifestyle changes. Set goals and adjust them based on your progress.

Did you know?

Room-temperature water digests better, but cold water forces your body to burn more calories to digest it.

"When you let your values guide your decisions, decision making becomes easier."

—Dr. Michael Olpin

"Finally, I am coming to the conclusion that my highest ambition is to be what I already am. That I will never fulfill my obligation to surpass myself, unless I first accept myself, and if I accept myself fully in the right way, I will already have surpassed myself."

—Thomas Merton

Values

IF YOU ARE an adult, think about what you enjoyed doing as a child, and ask yourself whether you are still doing these things today. Now, I know what you are thinking. You're thinking you are grown up, have a job and family, so you do not have time to enjoy the same activities. Maybe you are thinking that playing is for kids. Perhaps you are thinking you have grown out of that lifestyle.

"We don't stop playing because we grow old; we grow old because we stop playing."

I believe there is a lot of truth to this quote by George Bernard Shaw. For people to achieve great mental health, they need to continue to explore their passions, learn more, and try new things. It is only when we stop exploring and growing that we truly stagnate in life.

One of the core principles to achieving excellent mental health is to live a life according to your values. This is key to achieving a life of happiness and success. As simple as this is, it is amazing most people do not live a life according to their values. This is the source of a lot of problems in people's lives today with regards to their mental health.

We all make decisions every day. Some are little decisions, such as what are we going to eat for lunch, and others are major decisions, such as what career field to go into. Making decisions can be very stressful; often, we weigh out the pros and cons of each decision. When you let your values guide your decisions, making decisions becomes easier.

The first step is discovering what your values truly are. This requires you have an honest conversation with yourself and think about what you truly stand for as a person. An easy way to do this is to imagine you are at your own funeral at some point in the future. What would you want your friends, family, co-workers, and everyone who knew you to say about you? What would you want to be remembered for?

Those traits are what you should strive for in your life and the values that should guide your decisions. Ultimately, if we let our values guide our decisions, we will be happier and achieve the life we want to live.

Did you know?

Despite having the highest standard of living, Americans report having more mental health problems than other less-developed countries.

Overmedicated

ONE OF THE GREAT things about the United States is that we have the best access to high quality medication. Without a doubt, medication can absolutely be lifesaving at times. That said, Americans have become over-reliant on medications. In fact, Americans spend more money on medication per person than any other country, and yet the life expectancy in America is no higher than in other developed countries. Typically, doctors are very quick to prescribe a pill for problems, and most patients are happy to see their symptoms go away.

In many instances, though, drugs just mask the symptoms and do very little to help the body heal. For optimal healing to occur, we must discover the root cause of the disease, and this is something a drug typically cannot do.

For example, painkiller medication use and addiction to them are at an all-time high. These narcotic medications do nothing to help the body heal; they simply block the pain signals. Over time, more of the medication is needed in order to have the same effect, so it is very easy to become addicted to these toxic drugs. Furthermore, these powerful narcotic drugs are liver toxic and cause long-term liver damage. For this reason, America has a major narcotic drug addiction problem.

Without a doubt, there is a time and a place for medication. In some cases, medication can be absolutely life-saving. At the same time, prevention is always easier than curing. We should attempt to make the best choices possible to stack the deck in our favor when it comes to our health.

Because drugs can have bad side effects, we should make an effort to control our health through our lifestyle choices. Controlling your health through diet, exercise, sleep, relaxation, and minimizing toxins leads to true healing.

After all, there is no drug a person should want to be on for the rest of their life. When a doctor prescribes a patient a drug, there should almost always be a plan to eventually get that patient off the drug.

Did you know?

After alcohol, prescription drugs are the second most commonly abused drugs. Narcotic painkillers and attention deficit disorder medications are both highly abused prescription drugs. Many people use these prescription medications to get high.

"Never chase anyone. A person who appreciates you will walk with you."

—Author unknown

Social Health/Relationships

QUALITY RELATIONSHIPS are a vital part of our health and wellness. In general, the more connections we have with others, the happier and more successful we will become.

We should seek to enhance our relationships with others and develop relationships that are nurturing and improve our wellness. The following are essentials to developing positive relationships with others:

- ➤ Great communication, compassion, and understanding of others.
- ➤ Being honest and trustworthy with others.

- Understanding the personality of others and knowing how to best communicate with that individual.
- Knowing your own personality and biases that you may have.
- Being willing to compromise with others and seek out win-win opportunities.
- Taking on an assertive approach when dealing with others.
- Being kind and considerate to the needs of others
- Accepting people for who they are and tolerating all groups of people
- Not being afraid to develop relationships with people who have different interests than you

###

Did you know?

A long-term, eighty-year Harvard study showed that quality relationships are the best predictor of a long and healthy life.

Personalities

ONE OF THE BIGGEST misconceptions people have is that we tend to believe everyone thinks like us. Nothing can be further from the truth. Different people have different personalities.

To develop the best possible relationship with others, we must understand their personality. Knowing their personality is critical for communicating with them and developing a nurturing relationship.

Understanding the personality of others is important when communicating with them. For example, some people can handle sarcasm with a laugh and others are easily offended by it. While one comment may enhance your relationship with one person, it may weaken your relationship with another.

It is important that you take time to reflect on the personalities of those you are in relationships with. This allows you to communicate with them in a way that will enhance the relationship and not weaken it.

An example of different personality traits is the difference between introverts and extroverts. First, it is important to know that very few people are one or the other; most of us are blends of the two.

Introverts are people who get their energy from within. They like to think deeply, reflect, and analyze details. They are not quick to make decisions and often overthink situations. Because they listen more than talk, they are often mistaken as shy.

Extroverts get their energy from the outside world. They enjoy big events and small talk with others. They often make quick decisions and do not always think through decisions completely. An extrovert does not mind being the center of attention.

Having an awareness of where people fall on the introverted-versus-extroverted spectrum allows us to better understand and communicate with them. It is also important not to push people to take on a different personality. Part of developing good relationships with others is to accept people for who they are.

Did you know?

In her book *The Power of Introverts,* Susan Cain discusses the importance of introverts and how society tends to push people to be more extroverted.

Self-Awareness

WE ALL NEED to have an honest conversation with ourselves about our biases and weaknesses in our interpersonal interactions with others. Everyone has biases, and if we fail to recognize our own, they can lead us down the wrong path. Once we know our biases and admit we have them, we are more in control of ourselves and can prevent them from driving or interfering with our interactions with others.

Typically, we judge others based on our first impressions of them and then justify that judgment based on what happens after that. For example, if we judge someone to be a bad person, after that, we tend to see more of the bad in them than the good.

This can skew our view of others and wreck our chances at developing a strong relationship with that person.

Did you know?

Social intuition is the degree to which you can read the feelings of others in various social situations. People with great social intuition know the best way to respond to others in a situation.

Empathetic Listening

OFTEN, PEOPLE JUST want someone to talk to about their problems. If you find yourself in a situation where someone is communicating their distress to you, you can practice empathetic listening.

Empathetic listening is a technique we can use to show care, compassion, and empathy for someone who is communicating with us. The following are the different components of empathetic listening:

* Give them good eye contact while they are talking.
* Do not multi-task! Doing so will lead them to believe their concern is not important to you.

* Give them nonverbal cues of understanding such as a head nod to show them you are listening.

* Do not interrupt them! Let them talk, and wait for your turn to speak.

* When they are done speaking, ask clarifying questions or summarize what they told you. For example, "So my understanding is..." This gives them the impression you care.

* Do not feel you must immediately offer advice. It is okay to admit you are not sure of the best way to resolve their concerns or situation.

* Do tell them you feel bad for them and that they are on your mind.

When you use this technique, others will be appreciative of your willingness to help them. Many times, they just want someone to talk to, and oftentimes, the person will come up with a solution on their own. They may come to you more often and view you as someone they can trust.

Of course, not everyone likes to talk about their problems. We must be respectful of that, too.

Did you know?

Many times, people just want someone to communicate their problems or struggles with someone. Oftentimes, just listening to them empathetically will help them out.

Assertive Approach

HAVING AN ASSERTIVE approach when interacting with others is key. Being assertive allows you to communicate with others in an appropriate way when they have crossed into your "do not enter" territory. Being assertive is about not coming across as overly aggressive but, at the same time, not being passive. Being assertive is the best way to deal with confrontations with others and get the best results while not coming across as an angry lunatic.

The following are some examples of ways to take on a more assertive approach:

➢ Tell others when you are upset and why it bothers you.

➢ Admit when you are wrong, and apologize to others.

➢ Be willing to forgive others when they admit they were wrong.

➢ Be firm with your decisions, and tell others why you made them.

➢ Compliment others on their achievements and do not get jealous.

➢ Do not yell or shout; instead, talk in a confident voice tone.

➢ Talk over phone or in person when communicating something important.

➢ Always make decisions with your values in mind.

You will find that being assertive will make you a happier, more confident individual. Fewer people will try to walk over you. Best of all, you will be able to communicate your feelings effectively to others.

Did you know?

Being assertive will increase your chances of achieving inner peace. People who are too passive will not attain true inner peace, because their feelings get bottled up inside.

Kind Approach

A FAMOUS QUOTE by Maya Angelou states, "People will forget what you said, people will forget what you did, but people will not forget how you made them feel."

We should be as kind as possible to everyone! As the great Tom Shadyak says, humans function better in a state of kindness and empathy for others. Because of this, we should make it our fundamental goal to always be kind and considerate of others. (Note: that is not in SMART goal-setting format!!)

###

Did you know?

Research has shown that people who volunteer to help others live longer and are generally happier people. Continue to seek out ways to bring others up and make other people feel good about themselves.

Abusive Relationships

THE PURPOSE OF ANY relationship is to enhance your wellness. If the relationship is not improving your life, then it is time to get out.

The following are signs of an unhealthy relationship:

- ✓ Feelings of depression, guilt, or anxiety as a result of the relationship
- ✓ Cycle of verbal insults by the other person
- ✓ Someone is convincing you to do things against your values, morals, or ideals
- ✓ Physical or sexual violence
- ✓ Constant lying

Did you know?

On average, twenty-four people per minute are victims of rape, physical violence, or stalking by an intimate partner. That is nearly three in ten women and one in ten men who have experienced rape, physical violence, or stalking. 1-800-787-3224 is a National Domestic Violence hotline!

Diseases

YOUR HEALTH OUTCOMES are determined by your genetics and lifestyle behaviors. While it is true that some diseases are purely genetic, most diseases that plague Americans are largely due to lifestyle behaviors.

You have no control over the genes you are dealt, but you can do a lot to reduce your risk of chronic disease through your lifestyle choices. The leading cause of death among Americans today is heart disease, and the second is cancer. Other diseases that index highly among Americans are diabetes, osteoporosis, arthritis, and dementia.

###

Did you know?

Children born today are predicted to have a shorter life expectancy than their parents do.

Heart Disease

THE LEADING CAUSE of death in the United States continues to be heart disease. Heart disease has been called the silent killer because it is very progressive and, like many diseases, its symptoms are often not noticed in the early stages. In fact, a lot of people who suffer a heart attack never knew they had any cardiovascular issues.

Basically, our blood vessels distribute blood through the cells of our body. Blood contains oxygen, nutrients, hormones, and other things that are essential for life.

Atherosclerosis is the medical term for blood vessels being narrowed with plaque. This plaque can be the result of poor nutrition, lack of physical activity, and other lifestyle factors. As the blood vessels become narrower and narrower, there is an increased risk of a total blockage. That is when a heart attack can occur.

The following are tips to reduce your risk of cardiovascular disease:

- ➢ Eat a diet that is mostly whole, plant-based foods.
- ➢ Limit the amount of processed, packaged, and fast food you consume.
- ➢ Get at least thirty minutes of physical activity every day.
- ➢ Control your stress, as stress can cause plaque to build up.
- ➢ Get good quality sleep every night.
- ➢ Do not smoke or use electronic cigarettes, as both greatly increase your risk.

Did you know?

In the film *Forks over Knives,* the filmmakers show that atherosclerosis can be reversed by following a whole-food, plant-based diet. The body begins to repair itself!

Cancer

CANCER IS A DISEASE that many Americans continue to suffer from every day. While cancer is due partly as a result of one's genes, lifestyle can play a major causative role, as well.

Your body consists over a hundred trillion cells. Those cells need to repair and reproduce. Every day, your body produces millions of new cells. Several hundred to thousands of those cells are going to be cancerous. Your body relies on its immune system to not only recognize those cancerous cells but also to destroy them. Because of this, the immune system plays an enormous role in cancer prevention.

Because cancer is a disease of the cells, it can happen pretty much anywhere in the body. The most common of all cancers is skin cancer. Other common cancers include breast, prostate, lung, lymphoma, brain, blood, stomach, bladder, and liver cancer.

The following are tips for reducing your risk of cancer:

- ☐ Do not tan excessively or get sunburned. Use sunscreen, and wear layers when out in the sun.
- ☐ Eat a diet rich in fiber, and consume lots of plant-based foods.
- ☐ Limit the amount of processed, fast, and packaged foods.
- ☐ Do not smoke or use e-cigarettes, as they contain lots of carcinogenic chemicals.
- ☐ Maintain a healthy weight by getting plenty of exercise.
- ☐ Control stress, as stress weakens your immune system.
- ☐ Get quality sleep every night.

- ☐ Get regular medical check-ups.
- ☐ Learn how to self-check for breast (women), testicular (men), and skin cancer.

Did you know?

Skin cancer continues to be the leading cancer. Most skin cancers are harmless, but melanoma skin cancer is very threatening. One should look over their skin regularly and watch out for moles that are asymmetrical with irregular borders, color variations, and/or are large. Many dermatologists recommend the "ugly duckling" test. This means any mole that looks different from your other moles should be checked out by a trained physician.

Advertising

WE ARE CONSTANTLY bombarded with marketing and advertising everywhere we go. Companies are always trying to convince us that our lives will be better if we buy their product, whether it be a cup of coffee or a car. Advertising is really a nice way of calling what is really pure propaganda.

A variety of techniques are used by companies to deceive us into buying their products. Here are some of the common ones:

- Paying famous people millions of dollars to endorse their products and then using the celebrity's image to market.
- Promising fast results and then using images of before and after.

- Offering free gifts or a "buy now" discount.
- Using catch phrases.
- Using images and scenes that are pleasing to the eye.
- Attaching humor or a societal value to their product.

As obvious as some of these seem, it is important for us to be aware of these deceptive techniques as consumers. Before purchasing products, we must do our research and only buy products that meet our standards and make the most sense financially.

Did you know?

Corporations in the United States spend more money on advertising than the total economies of the 115 poorest countries.

Controversial Issues

IN THE FIELD of health, many controversial issues arise. When researching these issues and deciding your stance, it is important to consider different viewpoints, including science and your own personal values. Always remember that different experts can have entirely different opinions about these issues.

Here are some of the most popular controversial issues in health:

* Legalization of medicinal and recreational cannabis
* Is milk a health food?
* Should vaccinations be required?
* Is the vegan diet the best diet to consume?

* Are genetically modified crops harmful to the human body and environment?
* Should doctors be able to assist a patient with a terminal disease in a suicide?
* Should drug companies be able to advertise on television?
* Should companies be able to target children in their ads?

###

Did you know?

The website procon.org has information on controversial issues from many fields.

Sun Safety

SUNLIGHT HELPS our body produce vitamin D, which is vital for immune health and healthy bones. On the other hand, too much sunlight can be damaging to the skin, causing skin cancer, and aging the skin. To put it simply, you want to get some sunlight daily but not too much sunlight.

The following are sun safety tips:

- ✓ Be aware that the rays of the sun are strongest from mid-morning to late afternoon.
- ✓ After winter, your skin is not used to the sunlight and you are more likely to get

sunburned. Slowly acclimate your skin to the sun.

- ✓ Wear a hat and sunglasses and dress in layers, if you are going to be in the sun for a long time.
- ✓ If going to the beach or pool, seek shade. Alternate between a few minutes of sunlight and a few minutes in the shade.
- ✓ Wear sunscreen and reapply every few hours. Consider purchasing a mineral-based sunscreen that has fewer chemicals in it.
- ✓ Do not go into tanning salons, as they greatly increase your risk of skin cancer.

Did you know?

The darker your skin color, the longer sunlight exposure your skin needs to synthesize vitamin D. Light-skinned people can get adequate vitamin D in as little as twenty minutes of direct sunlight, while darker-skinned people need more sunlight. Unfortunately, the lighter your skin color, the higher your risk of skin cancer.

Concussions

CONCUSSIONS ARE VERY serious! Common ways to get a concussion include falling down on your head, getting hit in the head with a ball, or accidently hitting your head on something.

Common symptoms of a concussion include the following:

- Dizziness
- Headache
- Blurred vision
- Ringing in the ear
- Confusion
- Memory problems

If a person is involved in a fall, accident, or collision and has any of those symptoms, they need to take it very seriously, as those are signs they have suffered a concussion. It is important that the individual rest, recover, and seek medical attention.

Did you know?

The film *Head Games* is a great documentary covering the concussion crisis in America. It is worth watching!

Conclusion

THE FOLLOWING IS a list of the major points in this book:

- ❖ Your health can always can better or worse. It is constantly changing!
- ❖ Your body has an innate ability to heal itself, if you treat it right.
- ❖ Your overall state of wellness is the dynamic relationship between your physical, mental, and social health.
- ❖ Better health will lead to a better life!
- ❖ Fruit and vegetables are the keys to giving your body the nutrients it needs.
- ❖ Exercise can promote good mental and physical health.

❖ Toxins can harm your health! Do not smoke! Limit alcohol consumption!

❖ Quality sleep is essential to allow your body proper repair.

❖ Your thoughts and mindset are very powerful. Keep them positive!

❖ Set SMART goals to improve your health in any area that needs improvement.

❖ Your lifestyle choices can greatly reduce risk of chronic diseases.

###

I hope you enjoyed this book and found something to take away from it. Please do not hesitate to contact me at Ben.Mueller7@aol.com with any questions or requests for follow-up information.

With that, I wish you years of happy health. May all your goals and dreams come true.

Recommended Resources.

THE FOLLOWING FILMS and books taught and inspired me to formulate a successful strategy to living and feeling healthful and well. I encourage you to check them out!

Films:

Fat, Sick, and Nearly Dead

Fresh: New Thinking About What We're Eating

Hungry for Change

Forks Over Knives

Stress: Portrait of a Killer

Head Games

I AM

Books:

The China Study by T. Colin Campbell and Thomas M. Campbell II

Eat to Live: The Amazing Nutrient-Rich Program by Dr. Joel Fuhrman, M.D.

UnDo It! by Dr. Dean Ornish

Healing the Gerson Way by Charlotte Gerson

Unwind by Dr. Michael Olpin and Sam Bracken

Spark by John J. Ratey

The Paleo Diet by Loren Cordain, PhD

The Power of Introverts by Susan Cain

Attain Peak Running by Benjamin T. Mueller

Life's Operating Manual by Tom Shadyak

Omnivore's Dilemma by Michael Pollan

Glencoe Health by Mary H. Bronson and Don Merki

What Now

BEN IS AVAILABLE to do speaking engagements. Invite him to talk to your group about applying the principles mentioned in this book.

Please contact Ben through email at Ben.Mueller7@aol.com. He can do presentations varying from one hour to four hours, and each presentation can be tailored to meet your group's needs and interests.

About Ben

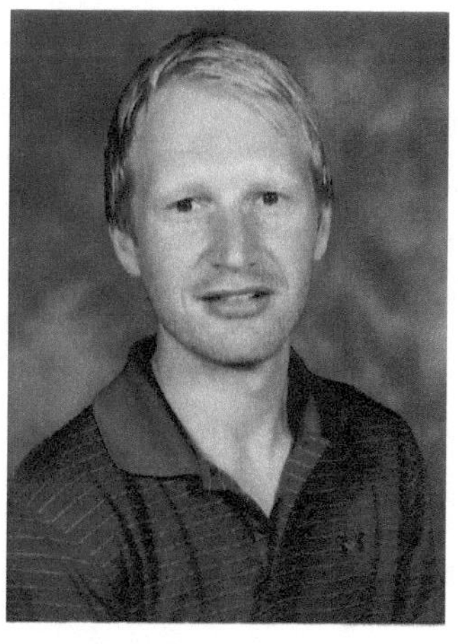

BEN MUELLER IS a wellness educator, endurance athlete, speaker, and activist. He has taught high school and junior college health and mathematics for over fifteen years.

Since he completed his first road race at the age of ten, Ben has not looked back. He is an avid runner and triathlete who has competed in over 500 road races, track races, and triathlons throughout the United States.

He qualified and competed in the United States national triathlon championships three times. He is also a Badger State Games (Wisconsin Olympics) gold medalist for multiple years in both the open and Masters categories.

Ben was born in Sheboygan, Wisconsin and went to college at UW-Whitewater. He earned his bachelor's degree in mathematics education and a master's degree in educational leadership at Concordia-Chicago. Currently, he is also a doctoral student for education at Concordia-Chicago, doing his doctoral research on exercise and its effects on coping with math anxiety.

When Ben is not training, he can be found refereeing soccer, rooting on the Wisconsin sports teams, or relaxing in a coffee shop.

Contact Ben here: Ben.mueller7@aol.com

Or find him here: BenjaminTMueller.webs.com

www.ingramcontent.com/pod-product-compliance
Lightning Source LLC
Chambersburg PA
CBHW051439250726
48655CB00001B/139